Trenton, Believe

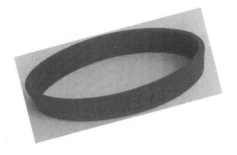

A mother's memoir of her son's recovery following an accident that leaves him a quadriplegic

BY SUSAN BAIER

TRENTON, BELIEVE

Published August 2016 by Susan Baier

ISBN-13: 978-1535545228

ISBN-10: 1535545224

TABLE OF CONTENTS

Dedications & Acknowledgements

2015 marks the tenth year since the accident which left you a quadriplegic; June 26, 2015, to be exact. I have wanted to write my thoughts for some time now, but I would start, and when it became too difficult, I would stop.

I am determined to forge through and compile my memories, the messages to you and the updates. For some reason that is yet to be proven, I feel a memoir of the past ten years would be helpful for you and me. I don't have to tell you how devastating this injury is. I hope this journal will provide awareness . . . awareness of the devastation this type of injury is to the person and the people surrounding you. If it is cathartic at the same time, I will take it. I am also hopeful it is cathartic for you as well.

I am certain you have little to no memory of the first three months after the accident. If you are like me you have very little memory of the first year of your injury. I believe the mind does this for a reason. The most painful memories are buried deep. Although I can't imagine anything more painful than what I do recall, I know these memories exist.

This documented journey is first and foremost for you. You are without a doubt the strongest person I know. You have shown strength, courage and fortitude in these past ten years. You surprise me daily with your sense of humor and kindness. I am so proud of you, and for that reason I want to honor you in this journey.

To Ashley and Jamie, your sisters, who provide you with normalcy. He is comfortable being himself with you. At times this can be hurtful, but you understand him. You are incredible sisters to him.

To Tyson, Ashley's husband, you are amazing. You are like a brother to Trenton and like another son to me. You provide friendship to Trenton and unconditional love to Ashley.

To Madison and Emma, Ashley and Tyson's daughters, you are our joy. We all love you so much. Trenton's face brightens when you walk in a room. Because you are nine and seven, you have never seen Trenton in anything but a wheelchair. When you saw the video of your Mom and Dad's wedding, it was the only time you have seen Trenton standing and walking. You were surprised by how tall he is.

To Chris, Jamie's husband, your passion is helping those with spinal cord injuries. I picked you from the beginning for Jamie. Thank God she smartened up and saw you as the rest of us did, an amazing individual.

To Liam, Chris and Jamie's son, you are a true joy. We cannot look at your face without feeling happiness and a sense of hopefulness.

To Rick and Cathy Baier, your father and stepmother, we certainly had our difficulties at first, but we have grown to love and respect one another. You have both worked hard to provide for Trenton and there is little doubt that the love we all have for him has brought us together.

To my sister Nancy, it is not easy living with Trenton. While you were in a position where financially it made sense, I know it is emotionally hard and physically difficult. I believe you have been good for each other and I thank you every day for taking on this endeavor.

To Ric 2, my boyfriend, you promised to stay by my side at the beginning and I know this has not been an easy promise for you to keep.

To my family and friends, thank you for sticking by me during the good and the bad. Your friendship and support are very important to me.

To Karen, my best friend since high school, you are my person. You listen to me, cry with me and allow me to be me.

To Sam, who lived with you for several years after your accident, you are without a doubt a fantastic person and a wonderful friend to Trenton. I don't know what we would do without you.

To Scott, another amazing and wonderful friend who has been by your side, not only throughout this journey, but a big part of your life.

To all of your friends who have been an important part of your life.

To all of our friends and family, it is a journey that has been made easier by your love and support.

Trenton, What Now?

Y ou had turned 24 and were celebrating at your Dad's lake house with a group of your buddies. I, too, was at the lake with Jamie, your younger sister, Sandy and Megan, longtime friends and neighbors. Megan and Jamie were to start college at the University of Missouri (MU) in the fall so we went to the lake for one night and the next morning our plan was to head to MU for new student orientation. As we often did, Sandy and I were talking that night sitting on her porch and having a glass of wine. We were discussing the divorce and I shared how I was concerned about you. I felt you were drinking too much and I had even told you this a few days prior to your heading to the lake for your birthday weekend. In your usual fashion you had blown off my comment, assuring me you knew what you were doing. This was not the first time you had assured me you knew what you were doing.

You were born on June 23, 1981. You came into this world somewhat ceremoniously, as you were born posterior (face up). My labor was not only difficult, but with every push I . . . well, let's just say it wasn't just you coming out of me. I can remember to this day

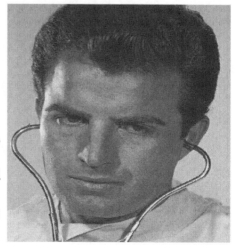

I didn't even want to push because my dilemma was being showcased by the big mirror at the foot of my bed. To make matters worse, there were several student nurses in the room and my doctor was exceptional looking. Honestly, you would have thought I would have been so consumed with the pain of the delivery, but all I could think about was everyone scrambling to find towels big enough to keep me cleaned up. I was so embarrassed, but being in the position I was, there was little I could do.

Finally, you were born. My first thought as I held you in my arms was how much I already loved you. My second was that I needed to find another OB/GYN . . . maybe one who did not look like Dr. Ben Casey from the hit 60s series. Need I say more?

You were an easy and happy baby. However, when you were six months old you were diagnosed with paroxysmal atrial tachycardia (PAT). I was trying to console you one cold January day and I could feel your heartbeat racing through your shirt. It was literally so fast I couldn't begin to count the beats. I immediately took you to the doctor and you were admitted.

PAT is characterized by a period of very rapid and irregular heartbeats that begin and end abruptly. The heart rate is usually between 160 and 200 beats per minute. The event would begin suddenly and end abruptly. You had Wolff-Parkinson-White syndrome, where some of your heart's electrical signals go down an extra or accessory pathway, which would cause your heart to race. From approximately six months on you took Digoxin, which kept your heart rate where it should be most of the time.

I also noticed when you were about three that one of your eyes wandered. We took you to the ophthalmologist, who informed us your vision was pretty bad. He was very abrupt with me and told me

I should have noticed your vision was bad sooner. He said, in words that would later be repeated in a slightly different version,

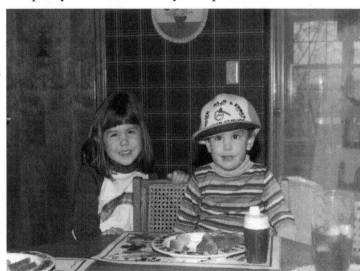

"Didn't you notice he couldn't see?" From the time you were three to about four we patched your eye, which eventually cured your lazy eye.

You were/are a great kid. You were somewhat lazy about certain things. School was definitely one of them. When you were in middle school you brought home your report card and you had a D in physical education (PE). I asked you how you could possibly get a D in PE. Of course you told me you had no idea. I called your teacher, who informed me you had not been dressing out. He explained he had sent a note home with you. Slightly frustrated, I asked your teacher if you weren't dressing out for PE did he really believe you would provide me a note telling me you weren't dressing out? I suggested to him that in the future it might be beneficial to call parents with this information a little sooner than the end of the school year. He agreed.

Funny story…many years later you received a phone call from the woman who had bought the house you grew up in. She had been cleaning out the attic and found a stack of notes you had hidden up there, as well as some test papers. I guess you started hiding them after I had told you the refrigerator door was where we put good test scores. I had gone in the kitchen one day and saw a test you had taped up with a "D" on it. We talked a little bit about what a good test score should look like. We never saw any more of your tests on the refrigerator.

While you never embraced school and studying, it was not for lack of trying on our part. Your dad and I tried bribes, money, things as a parent we never agreed with (which is why you never say "never" as a parent.) It didn't matter what we may have promised you because you were just not into the work. Mind you, we weren't asking for all As. But we knew you had much more potential and you were capable. What you did excel in was the social and sports aspects of school.

When your dad and I attended one of your high school parent/teacher conferences we were told you had gotten 8 out of 100 on a test. I looked at the teacher and said, "Well at least he got 8." Your dad nearly fell out of his chair. This is what it had become.

Kay, your teacher for your first class of the day, who is probably the most laid-back friend I have, had only one request: That you come dressed in the morning. You had her class first hour and you would get to class and then finish dressing. I really was concerned you would not graduate from high school, even though you had assured me you would. When we got to the graduation ceremony with Grandpa and Grandma and all your family, I quickly glanced at the program. I literally did not see your name at first and panicked. However, you did walk across that stage and received your diploma and then I panicked again, because I was thinking, NOW WHAT?

You were really a lot like me as a student. I was not interested in the academics of school, but I loved the social life. It is hard for me to understand this now, because I am definitely a Type A personality, and you think I would want to be good in everything, especially school. It also did not help, but certainly was not an excuse, that I lost my mom to breast cancer my ninth grade year in school. My dad was devastated. I felt so bad for him. He went to a movie by himself one night and it nearly broke my heart. But, being a teenager, and like most teenagers, I wanted to go out with my friends, etc.

When it was time to pick a college I didn't have a lot of choices. I wanted to go to MU, but I didn't have the grades. Karen, my best friend and who is now a Certified Registered Nurse Anesthetist and did care about grades, agreed to go to Northwest Missouri State University (NWMSU) with me. I loved it. I loved everything about it--the sorority, the partying, and being on my own. I seldom went to class and I would party the night before finals.

None of this am I proud of and later regretted it. It also didn't help, but again no excuse, that my freshman year in college and a week after my dad remarried, he passed away from a massive heart attack.

Nancy, my older sister, and I, were coming home for a celebratory party for Dad and Sue, his new wife. We pulled into the driveway and Jane, the oldest sister, was standing at the front door. I saw the look on her face and knew instantly Dad had died of something. He had been mowing the grass and collapsed. The neighbor boy tried CPR, but to no avail.

Poor Sue. She was from Tulsa, had never been married, had quit her job and moved to Kansas City, where she really didn't know anyone. She was wonderful. She did move back to Tulsa, which was completely understandable, and we still keep in contact with her. Jane and her husband, Dick, had married by then, so they became my guardians. They did their best, but for a girl who already was not that interested in getting an education, it was pretty much a given I would not finish college.

I met your dad in September of my freshman year at NWMSU. He was three years older, so I attended (if you could call it that) one more year and then the summer after your dad graduated we got married and moved to Iowa, where he taught school and coached wrestling and girls softball. So, while I understood you were unfortunately a lot like me, I did not want you to make the same mistakes I did. I wanted you to attend college and get your degree. I just couldn't do it for you.

Your plans after graduating from high school were to attend MU, but you didn't have the grades, so you opted to go to Maple Woods Community College, get your grades up and then apply to MU. During this time you got an apartment and worked for Dave, a good friend of mine, who owned apartments. You did maintenance work for the apartment complex. That didn't work out too well, as you

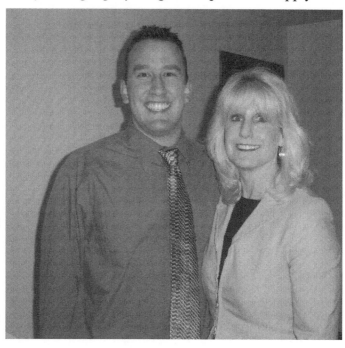

You and me on your college graduation day.

didn't do well at Maple Woods. Honestly, I'm not sure you ever went to class. Next, you decided you were going to go to a trade school and work at Budweiser. After working at Budweiser for a while, you thought maybe going to NWMSU would be a good idea. You got accepted, joined a fraternity, had a great time and did graduate.

It was a pretty good time in our lives. Your sister Ashley had met Tyson at MU and we loved him. She had graduated with her nursing degree from MU and landed a job at Liberty Hospital. They got married in October.

Jamie was a good student too and her plans were to also go to MU. Then your dad and I divorced. We had our justifications, but for some stupid reason I didn't feel it would have the impact on you all that it did. I was completely naïve. I can't change it and it does little good to talk about it, but I will always regret what I did to you kids.

June 26, 2005 Sunday, Lake of the Ozarks

So we went to the lake for one night, planning to head to MU the next morning for new student orientation.

About 2 a.m. my cell phone rang. I did not get good reception at the lake, so when I answered I could not understand what the person on the other end was saying. The phone went dead.

Instinctively, I knew something was terribly wrong. I got up and the phone rang again. I went outside, hoping I could hear the other person. It was your dad. He said you were in an accident, a bad accident, and you had been taken to the hospital at the lake. By this time, everyone was up. Sandy, Jamie and I threw on our clothes and we started driving. Sandy recently told me she had stopped a couple of times to make sure she was going in the right direction. I have no recollection of that. I do remember thinking it was taking forever and physically shaking, which was weird, because it was June and a warm night. The roads around the lake are windy and I get motion sick. I was nauseous, but unsure if it was nerves or the roads.

When we got to the hospital we saw your dad sitting on the curb with his head in his hands. I can still see his face and the look of total devastation. We got out of the car and he told us you were paralyzed and being flown to a Springfield, Missouri hospital. I don't remember much after that. Sandy told me later she kind of caught me as I seemed to be going down. I know Jamie was sobbing. I have no idea how long we stood there, but I am guessing not long, because I knew we needed to get on the road to Springfield. So I looked at Jamie and told her she needed to go with Sandy. I said everything was going to be alright and she needed to get registered for school. I still can't believe I did this to her. She was miserable, as she definitely didn't feel like going to MU. If this sounds weird to you, well it should, but I didn't want to believe what I had just been told. My way of dealing with it was to do what we were there to do, which was get Jamie registered for college. You were going to be fine and I needed to keep things normal. Sandy gave me a hug and her jacket, as I couldn't stop shaking.

Knowing you were on your way to Springfield, I wanted to get there as quickly as possible. Your dad told me he had to go back to the lake house and close things up. I was not real excited about this, but I was stuck, because I didn't have a car. I think your dad was in shock and not thinking, because I am pretty sure if he had been, we would have just headed for Springfield.

We didn't say much on our way back to his lake house, but I did ask him how this had happened. He explained you were all drinking by the hot tub and you had gotten up to cool off in the pool. You didn't come back, so thankfully Derek went to check on you and he found you face down in the pool. He pulled you out and did CPR. The ambulance was called, but it took 20 minutes for them to get there. I felt like I was going to be sick and I was sure at this point it was not the winding roads.

Many years later, when you talked about the accident, you said you did recall being in the pool and realizing you couldn't move. You were conscious briefly after being pulled out of the pool.

When we arrived at the lake house your friends were walking as if in slow motion. Literally everyone was moving at a snail's pace. I guess they were cleaning things up and gathering their stuff. I couldn't stand it, so I walked back outside and started pacing along the dock. I called my sister Jane, telling her I felt so helpless and that I was stuck. Of course, she had already heard. It is amazing how quickly the news got out. She told me to find someone who could take me to Springfield. I'm not sure how, but I did end up driving what I think was your car and your friend Scott came with me. We didn't talk much. For one thing, these kids were still drunk, on their way to a horrible hangover and, on top of that, a horrible nightmare was unfolding. I am the worst with directions and there wasn't GPS in the car. Truly, it is all such a blur, but somehow I got us to the hospital in Springfield, Missouri.

I had a lot of time to think in that car. All sorts of thoughts were going through my mind. Of course, I kept picturing Christopher

Reeve. Honestly, he was the only thing I could relate to when I heard the word "paralyzed." I wondered if it was true, and if you were paralyzed, would you want to live? I wondered if your dad had gotten catastrophic insurance, since you were 24 and didn't have a job yet. I prayed a lot.

When you were kids we went to church some and I had been raised in the Episcopalian Church. I did pray every night for the safety of my kids and friends and family, but I didn't go to church much. I wondered if God would even listen to me. I was mad at myself and thought somehow all of this was my fault. Had I not divorced your father, had I been stricter as a mother... you name it, I thought of it. I did attempt to call the hospital, but they wouldn't tell me anything. In the 2 to 2-1/2 hours it took for me to get there I had thought of everything.

Once we arrived and got to the intensive care unit (ICU), I was surprised to see nearly all your friends had made it before me. Everyone was sprawled everywhere. We had taken over the waiting room, kids lying on the floor; some were sleeping, but they all looked pretty rough. As I said, they had to sober up very quickly and I'm sure at this point they were feeling the effects of their hangovers. Family and friends arrived around the clock.

Ashley and Tyson picked up Jamie at MU (there was no way she could participate in orientation) and got stopped by the police for speeding on their way to Springfield. Ashley was crying so hard and trying to tell the officer what was going on. He gave them a warning, but told them they needed to slow down.

Cathy, your dad's girlfriend, (they hadn't married yet) and Ric 2, my boyfriend, (and called that because your dad is Rick also,) arrived. It was wonderful to have so much support and yet, so overwhelming. We hadn't even talked to a doctor yet.

Your dad and I were finally summoned by the neurosurgeon. He was a handsome man who looked at us with little to no empathy. I am pretty sure he saw the chaos and got a whiff of you and knew this was, yet again, an accident caused by alcohol.

He told us he would be performing surgery to basically keep your head from flopping around. Your neck was broken at the C-4-5 level. He said, "He will never walk again," adding that you would be paralyzed from the neck down.

I asked him if you knew you were paralyzed and I will never forget his response, "Well, if you woke up and couldn't move or feel anything, wouldn't you think 'I might be paralyzed'?" I didn't know if this man was in a bad mood or what his problem was, and I honestly didn't care. Your life was in his hands so I kept my thoughts to myself. I saw this same neurosurgeon right before we were leaving for Craig Hospital. He said in a disapproving tone, "So I understand you are looking into taking him to China." I had no idea where he had heard that. Sure, people had been talking about all sorts of places to go for treatment, but we were just trying to get you well enough to go to Craig at that point. I looked at him and said, "I will be forever grateful to you for saving my son's life, but if this was your son, wouldn't you do whatever you could to give him a chance at walking again?" He looked at me, gave me a nod and kept walking.

In preparation for your surgery a nurse by the name of Gary, who was much more compassionate, asked what medications you were taking, if any, and if you had any medical concerns they needed to know about. They also asked me if you had any tattoos, to which I replied in the negative.

We weren't able to see you before you went into surgery, so we walked out and let everyone know that surgery would involve securing the neck by putting a brace in with a screw on only one side. Surgery would be approximately 6-8 hours long.

At this point, phone calls were being made and more people were arriving. Your dad secured rooms at a Residence Inn nearby. I think most of us were operating on auto pilot. Families approached us in the waiting area, telling us they had been in our shoes just a few days ago and explained why they were there. This hospital takes a lot of the trauma cases that occur on the lake. During the summer months they see lots of boating accidents.

We spent your hours in surgery updating friends and family as more and more people arrived. There were so many people arriving around the clock that I wasn't able to think much while you were in surgery. This truly was a blessing.

Once surgery was over we were again summoned and told the

surgeon had successfully secured your neck. Again, this surgeon had done his job, and that was all we were going to get from him. I often say now that I would prefer a brilliant doctor over a compassionate one, but it would be nice if you could have both. Still, I will always be eternally grateful to this man.

The visiting hours for the ICU were 9-9:30 am, 1-1:30 pm, 4:30-5:00 pm and 8:30-9:30 pm. It was one big room with approximately 18 beds separated by curtain partitions maybe ten feet apart. There was little to no privacy and, whether you wanted to or not, you got to know why everyone was in there. If there was a new patient or a code, trauma or death, the visiting hour would be cancelled. You literally could wait all day and never get to see your loved one.

If it was hard for me to understand how critical you were, seeing you for the first time definitely made it real. You were intubated, so you couldn't talk. And, of course you couldn't eat. You also had a neck brace on. To my surprise, I saw that you had a tattoo--in fact, two of them. While you were pretty out of it and conversation was nearly impossible, I had to ask, "When did you get a tattoo?" I couldn't believe you had kept it hidden from me for so long.

When you were in high school, one of your buddies had been killed in a car accident. You were all coming from a party and following each other in your cars. It was a horrible time in your lives, and you had all decided to get a tattoo in his memory. When you first asked me about it, I had suggested you wait until you were older. Apparently, you didn't like my answer.

June 26 – July 19 in the Springfield, Missouri ICU

We stayed at the Residence Inn during this month. A lot of your friends stayed as long as they could and then would come back as often as they could. I literally only had the clothes I arrived at the hospital in. Angela, your cousin, offered to go by my house and pick up some of my things. I must have asked her to bring a certain pair of jeans. Because I still owned practically every pair of jeans I had since high school, she was a little confused as to which pair to bring. She showed up with about 20 pairs and thong underwear. I told her I didn't actually wear the thong underwear, just like I didn't wear most of the pairs of jeans I owned. And, out of all the jeans she brought, the pair I wanted was not in there. No biggie, just another excuse to go to Wal-Mart and walk around. As your stay in Springfield increased, there were times we just needed to get out of the hospital so Wal-Mart and Steve and Barry's were our go-to places.

As I mentioned, the news of your accident had traveled around very quickly. A lot of what was being said was not accurate or even close to being accurate. For example, your friend Chris was supposedly so depressed he was on suicide watch. Actually, Chris was completely exhausted and nearly passed out from that and the stress. Another one of your friends, Sam, supposedly had gotten so sunburned he had to see a doctor. He was sunburned and was using his Aloe Vera cream, but he had left it in the waiting room and the cleaning crew had thrown it away.

Because we wanted our friends and families updated with accurate information, we started doing daily updates. My friend Linda would initially provide the updates and then, when we got to Colorado for rehabilitation, I took over.

Our routine was pretty much the same every day. We would get up and get ready to spend the day at the hospital. We would get there in time for the morning visiting hour. After that, some would go back to the hotel or maybe make the run to Wal-Mart, but typically we stayed at the hospital. Thankfully my family stepped in and took charge of things I couldn't even think of.

My sister Jane was instrumental in researching rehabilitation facilities. We wanted to get you moved as soon as you were stable enough. She was also taking care of my dogs (two Shih Tzus) while I was in Springfield. They were puppies I had just brought home so they weren't even potty-trained yet.

Lindsay, my niece, had connections in Washington D.C. and was hoping to contact a physician who specialized in cases of paralysis.

Rick had purchased catastrophic insurance for you, but we needed to get you on Medicare. I couldn't begin to think about any of that. You were still quite critical and my focus was on you.

Friends and family would come for the day delivering food and goodies. The next visiting hour would come and we would see you and then wait for the evening visiting hour.

As you can imagine, the stress of your injury, plus the family dynamics, caused some pretty rough moments. We were all together pretty much 24/7. Our divorce was pretty new. While everyone, including me, had met Cathy and the same with Ric 2, we were suddenly put into a situation where we saw each other every day. I know this is going to come as a shock to you, but we are not a perfect family. We had our fights and disagreements and they were not always private. But when I look back at that time and that situation, I think we did pretty well. Bottom line, we were all there for you and we were all handling the situation the best we could.

Ric 2 was a snorer, and a loud one. We were packed into these hotel rooms. Sleeping was a problem. Someone had managed to get me some sleeping pills, so I typically crashed. Jamie, on the other hand, had a terrible time with Ric's snoring. She could hear him whether she was sleeping on the other double bed or on the couch outside the room. She would walk the halls in tears from exhaustion.

Ric's shoes also stank, whether he was wearing them or not. At first we could not understand why they would smell so bad, but realized it must have been because he wasn't wearing socks with them. Of course we laughed about it, but I finally told him he was going to have to throw them away. Back to Steve and Barry's we went, where Ric 2 bought a new pair of shoes and lots of extra socks. Ric 2 also started a journal and began writing down names of everyone that came to visit you, as well as what went on each day you were in Springfield. I am so thankful he did, because as I mentioned earlier, your mind has a way of blocking things from your memory. And many of the following stories I had not remembered.

Journal Notes

June 28, 2005 Tuesday

On this day you had a procedure to help prevent blood clots. It was called an Inferior Vena Cava Filter placement. An inferior vena cava is a large vein that carries deoxygenated blood from the lower body to the heart. A radiologist uses image guidance to place a filter in the inferior vena cava. Blood clots that develop in the veins of the leg or pelvis occasionally break up and can travel to the lungs. This filter traps the fragments and prevents them from traveling to the vena cava vein to the heart and lungs. Years later you developed a blood clot and these notes helped us to remember you had this procedure.

There were still a lot of people in Springfield and, contrary to what the surgeon had said, you had not figured out you were paralyzed.

We were also told a prayer service was arranged for friends and families at St. Charles Church in Kansas City on June 28. For those of us who were in Springfield, they taped it. It would not be until you got to Colorado that you would be able to watch the tape. We were all so grateful for the outpouring of prayers and support.

While most of the patients in the Springfield ICU were from the lake and accidents on the lake, we met a family whose child had been in a motorcycle accident and another one had been in a car accident. The boy in the motorcycle accident lost an arm and a leg. The younger boy who had been in the car accident would improve and then decline and eventually pass away. It truly was heartbreaking. There is an instant bond with these families. You understand their pain and they understand yours. During this time we lived and breathed the ICU. Even if we tried to go somewhere or do something different, it was impossible to stop thinking about you.

There are so many emotions that occur when you first hear of a loved one's accident/illness. My initial reaction was shock and then very quickly it turned to fear. I was fortunate to have family that offered to help at home with the dogs etc. Because I had this support I could concentrate on you.

My supervisors at Children's Mercy Hospital (CMH), which is where I worked and still do, were also incredibly gracious and accommodating. Since your accident, and now that I work as a patient advocate at CMH, I see families that don't have this support. While it is never easy, it does help to have family closeby and an employer who understands and is willing to work with you and your family.

June 29, Wednesday (Realizing you are paralyzed)
It is now three days after the accident. Having a conversation with you was extremely difficult, tedious and frustrating for you and confusing to us. If you could answer a question with yes or no it was pretty simple; you just nodded or shook your head. But you had questions for us. So I would start with the letter "A" and go through the alphabet. You would nod when I got to the letter you wanted and we spelled out the word or words that way.

During one of our visits I started going through the alphabet a, b, etc. and got to "N" then a, b and got to "U" then a, b and got to "M" and then a, b and got to "B". You had spelled out "numb." I asked you if the surgeon had told you much and you shook your head. I asked if you wanted to know and you nodded yes. I remember I did not want to mention the word "paralyzed" and was glad you had spelled numb. I said, yes, you are numb, but that we were looking at rehabilitation and options to help you. I know at the time it was one of the worst moments of my life. I can only imagine how difficult it must have been for you.

So now you know and you are scared. You have a lot of questions as to what will happen next. We talk a lot about getting off the vent because initially we were told we couldn't move you to another facility to start rehabilitation until this occurred. I know we must have put a lot of pressure on you because we felt pressured. It was like something magical would happen if we could get you to Craig Hospital in Englewood, Colorado. On top of that, you developed pneumonia. When you were found in the pool you were face down, so we weren't necessarily surprised by this news; however, it was still a setback and very disheartening.

Update from Linda

Thank you for attending the prayer service last night. Those who could not attend, I know that you were thinking of Trenton. Trenton's condition is basically the same, but he has also developed pneumonia. He is aware of what is going on and is very, very scared. The good news (finally) is that they have a contact and the names of other doctors in this field that may be of help to Trenton (one I believe had treated Christopher Reeve).

Let's hope and pray that every day will bring a little more good news.

Update from your Dad

Trenton was pretty out of it yesterday due to him now realizing his problem. Through the efforts of my niece (Lindsay) who works on Capitol Hill in Washington DC, she has put us in contact with the personal physician and best friend of Christopher Reeve. He has agreed to review Trenton's case. If he meets all criteria we will move him to a location where they are conducting new research and procedures. I have a conference call with him today. It is a miracle that we have pulled this off, thanks to Lindsay. Thanks for your support and prayers. I will probably not be back this week, but feel free to call and I will try to get back to you. Just keep doing deals and if I do not talk to you, enjoy the holidays with your families

We were all encouraged with the opportunity to work with Christopher Reeve's doctor, Dr. John McDonald, even though I don't think we had a clue what that meant. We were coming to a close of the first week of the accident. Many of your friends were still with us at the Residence Inn. I guess we were in somewhat of a routine at this point. Food was arriving around the clock and our friends and family came in for an hour or to spend the day with us. Conversations with Craig had begun and a woman from Craig was scheduled to fly in the following Wednesday, July 6, for evaluation. We were all so hopeful this would work out.

So, our days were pretty busy with little time to think, but then the evenings would come around and they were brutal. Pretty much the only alone time I had was when I took a shower. I broke down a lot in the shower and cursed the world. I was not, and am still not, a big crier in public. I felt like I needed to be in control, which is how I have always dealt with things. I was also trying to be strong and positive for Ashley and Jamie. They were struggling and your dad was not doing well. I know he was blaming himself. This was not his fault. It was what it was--and while I wanted to be positive, it was very difficult to feel positive about anything at this point.

July 3, Sunday

Your friends were sitting around and joking about cooking with you. I didn't know you cooked much, so was once again surprised by all the things I was learning about you. Ashley, Jamie and I went to the t-shirt shop to get the $5.98 t-shirt and pajama bottoms, per Yvette's (your nurse) request. Several of your friends were heading back to Kansas City and told you "See you later." When the 4:30 visiting half hour arrived, the doors actually opened at 4:30. This never happened. You were in your new clothes and looked good. Yvette said she had given you a bath and shaved you. She told us she had a great conversation with you. You had told her about Willy, your dog, and she was telling you her dog went to day care. Yvette told us she really liked you and had a cute little sister your age. She then told us you got a big grin on your face. You weren't real talkative when we were visiting. I think your bath, etc. had worn you out. Yvette told me she was sorry she had gotten all the quality conversations. I told her I didn't care, and that I was just glad you were talking (mouthing would be a better way to put it). I asked you if you wanted to sleep and we would come back later. You opened your eyes and gave me a big smile and mouthed, "Yes."

It was hard not hearing your voice, so I started calling your cell phone so I could hear it. I knew it was stupid, but it helped.

July 4, Monday

You were wide awake for the morning visiting hours. You had a lot of questions and asked when the woman was coming from Craig to evaluate you. You also asked what they do at Craig. I explained to you they would wean you off the ventilator and there would be rehabilitation. Originally, we had been told you couldn't be on the ventilator when you were moved, but later we were told you could, which was good news. It was definitely less pressure for you. You were still dealing with pneumonia in one lung so we had to get you well before you could travel.

Derek's parents (he pulled you out of the pool) were taking care of your dog Willy and Derek's cousin had brought you a picture of Willy, but you were too tired last night to look at it. We showed you the picture this morning and you smiled. You then looked at me and gave me a really BIG SMILE that lasted for about five seconds. I told you how much that made my day.

The 1 p.m. visit was the best so far. The doors opened at 1:16 pm and you were wide awake. Larry and Judy (longtime friends and neighbors) visited. Larry had sweated through his shirt walking into the hospital and his shirt looked like Mickey Mouse ears. We were there for about 35 minutes when you said you didn't want us to leave, but you needed to rest. I read several cards you had received and your dad told you the Royals had lost. I told you that you had been "Googled" and that your dad had been rear-ended on his way to the hospital.

July 5, Tuesday

They were two hours late opening the doors. We were pretty sure it was because of you. When we did get into your room you told us you had an operation. They had put a tube in to drain fluid from your lungs. You were still running a fever. You were very talkative and did not want us to leave. You said you wanted to go to Denver tomorrow! We explained how long you might be there. Your pants were off and you had the hospital gown back on. You smiled because you knew they had to throw the pants away because you had a big poop.

I realize some of the things written here could be embarrassing to you. This is definitely not my intent. I do think it is important for anyone reading this to understand the depth of this injury. The only way to raise awareness is to be honest about the effects.

Journal Notes - July 6, Wednesday

You had a good night, according to your nurse, Jason. You told us it was just ok. You were in the chair and you did not like the chair, so you were kind of grumpy. You were told you were going to have a tracheotomy (an incision in the windpipe forming a temporary or permanent opening) today and you were somewhat anxious about it. When we visited at 1:00 you were much better. You wondered where your car was. I explained the trach and how it was not permanent. We talked a lot about Colorado and what you would be doing. You asked if you could do commercial real estate. Your dad was a commercial realtor and you had hoped to work with him one day. You wanted to know how we were paying for all of this. Jamie was upset because she didn't think you were being nice to her because you didn't smile at her. Of course you had no idea how much we all relied on that smile. You then told us you had lost a tooth in the accident. Sure enough, it was gone. You showed us it was missing several times during that visit.

Our entire day was focused around the ICU and their visiting hours. The doors would open and in we would go. On one visit, I walked up to the bed and patted your hand only to find out I had not walked far enough. The dad of the patient whose hand I was patting was laughing. I was so embarrassed. One of your friends had done the same thing with the same patient at another visit.

The representative from Craig did not come today as we had originally been told, and would be in Springfield on Friday.

Journal Notes - July 7, Thursday

You were very chatty during the morning visit. You mouthed you felt badly for Chris, who had just gotten an apartment with you. Jamie and I told you not to worry about it. You asked Jamie and me if we wanted to stay and watch TV while you napped. We loved when you would ask us to stay. Susie, Allison and Ryan, longtime friends, were at the 1:00 pm visit. You were glad to see them. You were telling everyone you had swallowed your tooth. Stella, your nurse, came in to prep you for your trach. When the procedure was finished we came back in and you looked good. I was able to give you sips of apple juice and Jell-O, plus we could read your lips better.

The 8:30 visit was late because someone in the ICU had passed away. You were in your chair and tired of being in it. Chris and Erin, his girlfriend, were back and you were glad to see them. Ric 2 went home and Jamie and I were going home tomorrow. I was of course worried about leaving you, but you told me you would be ok.

During this time we were also working with the complex where you and Chris had literally just moved into. The realization was you would not be able to move back in with Chris in the apartment. Thankfully, we knew the manager of the complex so he worked with us and let Chris stay there for a couple of months.

I had gone back to Kansas City for a weekend so I went to the apartment and got your clothes. To say this was another one of the most difficult times of my life is an understatement. I probably should not have gone by myself, but I don't think I could have done it any other way. I laid on your bed thinking about you as a little boy and your school years, the struggles with finding what you wanted to do in life and you finally figuring it out, and now it was gone. I wanted to go back in time and do something different, though I didn't know what I could change so you wouldn't be where you were now. I had never felt that kind of sadness before, the sadness of a parent's inability to fix or help their child.

Craig Hospital, here we come... wait a minute; not so fast

July 8, Friday Update from Linda

Trenton is in great spirits today. He is very animated and relaxed. Trenton's white count is high and he has an infection. The Craig Institute representative visited today and decided that Trenton would leave for Denver Tuesday, July 12. The rep was very good with him and explained that a tracheal tube would be inserted and also discussed with him the aspects of his breathing and really put him at ease. He will also continue to be heavily medicated before the trip. She also said upon completion of rehab (no time frame) he will be able to do more things than not. She expects that he will only need help in the morning and the evening and be pretty self-sufficient. Susan and Rick have yet to coordinate their plans, but Susan believes that she will return home for a few days before driving to Colorado.

So many of you have asked where to send cards, etc. and what you can do. The family continues to ask for your prayers and suggests that you probably wait until they are in Denver for cards, etc. I suggested that those who live locally could stop by and help her get ready to leave. I'll let you know if there are things for us to do. Don't hesitate to contact Susan to ask about visiting, Trenton's condition, etc.

As I read this update ten years later stating you would be able to do more things than not and you would only need help in the morning and in the evenings, I would mostly agree. The technology today allows you to control your heat. You can turn on and off your lights, fan and control your television. We are working towards getting you a device which will allow you to control the door that goes into your garage. On nice days you like to sit outside. You have a television in the garage as well. You have Dragon voice recognition software on your computer, which allows you to do what the rest of us can do. It may just take you a little longer to do it. Your caregivers get you ready in the morning and fix lunch and then they are back in the evenings to get you to bed. Nancy does dinner.

Sounds pretty simple in writing, but it is the exact opposite of simple. Everything you do requires planning. You need someone to drive you. You have to think about where you are going. For example, your dad lives at a lake. The hill going down to the dock is very steep. If it rains, it is nearly impossible to get you down the hill. You have tipped over once and hit your head on a rock. Your dad can't put in a sidewalk due the neighbors' sprinklers. This last time you were there I brought a bunch of cardboard and we lined the trail with cardboard and it still took three to four people on each side of you to ensure you didn't tip over again. To get into someone's house you have to have zero entry, meaning there isn't a step. So we have to have a ramp to get you into most houses. You have been stuck in mud and snow before. The world is not as wheelchair-accessible as we think. Every building I go into now I look at totally from your perspective and am shocked that most are difficult for you to access.

July 10, Sunday Update from Me

Hi all,

Trenton had his trach done today about 1:30. We got to go in to see him a couple of hours later and he was sitting in his chair and drinking some apple juice from a straw and I fed him a couple of bites of strawberry Jell-O. He did pretty well. I imagine it will take some time to get used to it, but he said it felt a whole lot better. We can understand when he mouths things better and he is very chatty. I can see no reason why he won't be leaving for Colorado early Tuesday morning. I know there will be bumps in the road but his attitude seems amazing. Thanks for all your love and support and I will keep you posted.

Update from Linda

I forwarded everyone an e-mail from Susan yesterday. She plans to be home sometime this weekend. She asked me to keep my e-mail listings and updates open until she has the time to coordinate a few lists that are circulating, so I will continue to keep you updated and also forward her mail to you.

I believe that the current plan is that Rick will fly to Denver with Trenton and Susan will return home for a few days and leave for Denver next Friday. I know that she has a lot of arrangements to make, because once in Denver she will return home for short periods of time.

I thought that many would like to see Susan before she leaves, but are hesitant to call or visit. I have reserved the back room of Tommy's next Wednesday, July 13, from 5:30 p.m. on (maybe until 8:00?) Anyone who would like to drop by and see Susan is welcome.

Come by for five minutes or two hours, I think that she would enjoy seeing everyone.

Linda had invited my friends to meet at a restaurant while I was home from Springfield and before I went to Denver. It was wonderful to see my friends. And, if I am being completely honest, it was somewhat exhausting. I was trying so hard to stay strong and appear normal when I clearly was not. Still, I was very appreciative of the support.

July 12, Tuesday Update from Linda

Trenton has had to have the feeding tube reinserted in his abdomen because the feeding tube through his nose proved to be too painful. Trenton and Rick will not be able to make the trip to Denver today. The Craig Institute does not currently have a space for Trenton and has indicated that it could be 7-10 days before one is available. Susan plans to leave for Springfield Thursday and possibly leave for Denver from there. Susan is devastated by this latest turn of events. Hopefully our prayers will guide him there sooner.

July 17, Sunday Update from Linda

Trenton is doing great. He has a great attitude and has set some goals for himself. He is working so very hard to be independent from the ventilator. Susan said that he is at 5 and when he reaches 0 he is off! He is having long and detailed discussions with everyone and is ready to be on his way. He has been somewhat anxious and the ICU has allowed the family to spend the night with him. Tuesday is still the departure day and we even have a time...9:30 am.

During this time it was a constant roller coaster. We so wanted to get you to Craig, but things kept coming up. It was hard on everyone. I know it was incredibly hard on you. Your anxiety was very apparent. I was unaware of how much medication you were on, but soon learned how you reacted to Morphine. At this point, you had been moved to another ICU (less intense, so to speak) and could have people with you around the clock. They had put you in a bed that oscillated for preventing pressure ulcers.

The nurses had no problem with us staying with you 24/7. I think you were somewhat of a handful. You had lots of questions, fears and irrational thoughts. We were more than happy to stay with you. You were saying (again mouthing) some pretty bizarre things and making me nervous. For starters, you were sure the staff was trying to kill you. You didn't want to be alone and would say, "Mom, they are trying to kill me in here." There was no convincing you otherwise.

Ashley was in the room chatting with you when you looked at her and said, "Ashley, quit touching the nurse's vagina." She asked you, "What nurse?" You said, "The nurse standing right next to you." Ashley looked around and said, "Trenton there isn't a nurse in here and even if there was, I wouldn't be touching her." You said, "She is right there and quit touching her." You were dead serious and it was a little scary. But, we also couldn't help laughing at times.

Everyone was engulfed in constant stress, sadness and fear and occasionally someone would say something amusing. Even if it wasn't that funny, it felt good to laugh. I had no idea how much Morphine you were on, but apparently this was the cause of the hallucinations and bizarre thoughts.

You explained to me when reading this book that part of your anxiety during that time was hearing the Code Blue announcements in the hospital. This makes complete sense and is probably why some hospitals no longer do Code Blue overhead announcements!

July 19, Tuesday Update from Linda

I know that we are all waiting anxiously to hear that Trenton is in the air and on his way to Denver. As of 10:00 a.m. the Craig Institute people had not arrived. As wonderful as his attitude has been, Trenton has been extremely anxious and nervous and has had trouble sleeping the last few days. The anticipation of this trip has been difficult for him. As soon as Susan calls with the news that Trenton and Rick are in the air, I'll let you know.

Craig Hospital, Finally

July 19, Tuesday Update from Linda

Trenton is settling in at the Craig Institute. He has a private room that includes a section that has a refrigerator, pullout bed and other amenities. The Institute is connected to the Swedish Hospital where the testing is done. The apartment where Rick and Susan will be staying is situated within steps of the entrance to the Institute. The staff wears shorts and t-shirts! The Institute is only a 55-bed facility.

Trenton is spending much of his time being examined and evaluated. I don't think that they have completed this and I have not heard of any results. Trenton is actually in rehab already. He has physical and occupational therapy daily and will have speech therapy when he is off the ventilator. He was off the ventilator for 12 minutes yesterday and spoke a few words. Rick is really impressed with Trenton's doctor. He said that he has a great sense of humor.

Susan left this morning for Denver and plans to arrive this evening. She probably won't touch base with us until tomorrow at the earliest. Today and tomorrow will be very full days for her. Rick is returning to Kansas City late this evening.

I called the Institute this morning and anything can be sent to Trenton. Rick will receive the apartment information this afternoon, which will include the direct telephone number.

I drove to Englewood, Colorado on Tuesday, July 19. Your Dad had flown with you in the medical plane. You had done well during the trip. When I arrived at Craig your Dad showed me around the facility. I honestly wasn't all that interested because I wanted to get back to you, but the place was very impressive.

Craig Hospital was originally founded by Frank Craig in 1907 to treat indigent men with tuberculosis. It later became known for treatment of spinal cord injuries (SCI) and traumatic brain injuries (TBI). Their research department is devoted to rehabilitation of SCI and TBIs.

After our tour your Dad headed back to KC and I went back to your room. I had been there less than five minutes when all the bells and whistles attached to you went off (Code Blue). Staff ran in and I stepped outside to the hallway right in front of your room. I had no idea what had happened. In the five minutes I had seen you, you had seemed just fine. A woman I didn't know started talking to me and telling me it was going to be ok. I was told by someone years later that while everyone was working on you, you looked out to the hallway and you saw the look on my face. You had told them you never wanted to see that look on my face again

I have no idea how long it took, but eventually you were ok and I could come back into your room. I believe your tracheal tube had become dislodged, causing the respiratory distress.

Once I knew you were ok, I really needed to unravel by myself. I didn't want to do this in front of you so I thought it would be a good time to get my stuff to my room where I would be staying. You said you were ok with this so I walked over to the apartments or rooms. It was not far. I didn't want to cry on my way over so I tried not to make eye contact with anyone. I was walking quite purposefully to the room, got my key and let myself in. It was then that it all hit me. I think I wanted so much to believe this was not all real.

The room was large and completely wheelchair-accessible. I was a little confused at first because I knew you wouldn't be able to stay with me. I understood later the patients who come back for checkups and don't require being inpatient stay at the apartments. I took my stuff and unpacked a little bit. I really wasn't in the mood to get "settled in."

Jane had contacted a doctor right after the accident to get me some anti-depressants. I didn't want to take them and honestly thought I could do this without taking them. But I gave in and dug for them in my bag and popped one in. I knew I could not be a blubbering mess around you and that I would not be doing anybody any good if I didn't get control of myself.

The staff at Craig was amazing. I cannot say enough good things about all of them. They were kind, warm, honest and informative . . perhaps a little too informative. I literally got enough Spinal Cord

Injury information to fill a king size comforter box. It was too much. I tried to read it, but it put the fear of God in me as to what could go wrong. I pretty much knew instinctively what could go wrong. I figured they were going to go over most of it anyway. Maybe this was me being in denial, but I couldn't do it. I couldn't read it and to this day I still have not read it.

Sometimes when you were sleeping I would pinch your leg or foot to look for a reaction. You would wake up occasionally and ask me what I was doing. I told myself you woke up because you could feel it. Unfortunately, this was not the case, but rather the intense pinching would cause a spasm. I also sprinkled holy water on you that Gloria, the mother of one of your friends, gave me. You were a good sport and allowed me to do this.

When you kids were young we really did try to go to church on a regular basis. You had been baptized, confirmed and even sang in the church choir. I knew my faith had been rocked with your accident and, while we hadn't talked about it, I wondered about yours. I wanted to believe, but sometimes it was just too hard. I had several people say to me during this time, "You know, God only gives you as much as you can handle." Or, "You are so strong, I could never handle this." I wanted to say, "Are you fucking kidding me? Do you think I can handle this and no, I am not that strong." I also had a few people say to me, "Oh, he must have been drinking." Of course he was drinking, you moron. Who dives into a shallow pool sober? I know no one meant to say those things viciously and again, on a better day, none of this would have bothered me. But they were not good days and it did bother me.

The news is out and emails from friends and family start coming in

July 20, Wednesday, Email from Allison (your high school friend).
Hi Susan, It's Allison. I got your email address from my mom's addresses. I just wanted to write because I didn't know how else to get in touch with you guys and Trenton. I heard that Trenton will be finally going to Colorado on Tuesday, and that is great news. I also hear that he is doing great weaning off the ventilator; also great! I am still praying for you guys and thinking about Trenton daily, if you would let him know that. I also never take his bracelet off, as it is a reminder daily to continue to pray for him. I hope he is keeping his spirits up. I was pleased when I saw Trenton because I saw in his eyes his spirit and his great contagious smile. Mainly I just wanted you to know I was thinking of all of you, but for you to please let Trenton know that I am thinking about him. Continue to take it one day at a time, and stay strong, as I know all of you will.

Right after your accident your Dad had bracelets made similar to the "Live Strong" bracelets. Yours were blue and we used the word "Believe." Your Dad and I wear ours still today and so does Karen. In fact, Karen, who goes to Haiti every year with the eye team for missionary work (she performs the eye blocks), had the bracelet on and a Haitian boy took an interest in it. She gave it to him and of course, I provided her with a new one.

July 24, Sunday, Email to Jane (my sister) from me
Trenton has still been very nauseous today. It is a little frustrating

for him, but they are trying to figure out what is causing it. I really am doing fine. Diane, a friend of mine who happened to be in Denver, brought me a sandwich, salad, cookies and M&Ms on her way back to Kansas City. It is just very hard to leave him right now. Tomorrow he starts his therapy and hopefully will feel better, although I think that every day. It will be good when Jamie gets here, then Ric 2 will fly out and drive back with me, so I will be fine. Thanks for everything and I know you and Nancy would do anything for me. Just not a lot anyone else can do right now. I will let you know how tomorrow goes. Thanks again.

My email to Sue (Your step-grandmother)
Hi Sue,

Thanks for your note. We are in Colorado and things are going ok. He has been sick for about four days as he has so much junk in his lungs. He is better today and rested well last night and this morning. He is going to get up this afternoon and go to physical therapy. They are waiting a bit to totally wean him from the ventilator because of his lungs being so full. However, I really don't anticipate that to be too much longer. I am with him 24/7 as he has been so nervous, scared and anxious. I am hanging in there, thanks to drugs. I should be stronger but this is bigger than I am. I am trying to be strong but we are all struggling. I will be here through the 8th of August and then head to KC to get Jamie off to MU and stay and try to work a few weeks and then back here for a while.

July 26, Tuesday, Email from Allison
Hi Susan... I hope you don't mind me emailing you. I don't know how else to let Trenton and all of you know that I am thinking about you guys. How is Trenton? Are the anxiousness and ventilator settings coming any better? Being nauseous is the worst feeling; it's got to feel scary being weaned off the ventilator, but I know Trenton can do it. The hard work starts tomorrow for Trenton. Let him know how strong I know he is and to think positive thoughts, plus take it one day at a time. How are his spirits along with yours and Rick's?

Craig Hospital is an amazing place from what I've read....there couldn't be a better place for Trenton's rehab. I hope I can talk to

Trenton on the phone soon after he gets weaned off the vent. I will definitely be in touch often. Tell Trenton that those nurses and staff in Colorado better be taking good care of him, or else his nurses in KC (Ashley and I) are gonna be raising hell (haha).

I don't think I ever told Trenton about my puppy, so you'll have to tell him. Maybe I'll send a picture. My puppy, Cooper, is doing well. He can roll over now and sit. There still have been accidents in the house when he gets excited or I'm not paying enough attention to him. How old are your puppies? I don't mind babysitting your puppies if you ever need me to on one of my four days off a week. They might actually play and keep Cooper occupied. Just let me know. I remember when Trenton had his puppy in high school and it was small enough to fit in his coat pocket!

I also wanted to let you know that I am working on Jamie's recommendation letter to Pi Phi, so it should be in the mail this week.

Stay positive and don't forget how many people are praying for you, Trenton, and your whole family. I definitely am. I will keep in touch, and please feel free to share any of my emails with Trenton. I'm sure he likes hearing from KC. I wasn't sure if you remembered me telling you about "Care Pages" that the Craig Hospital website offers. The page is like a webpage that you guys can put info on and others can write on too. I didn't know if you guys were going to use that or not. Just let me know so I can access it if you do.

Trenton, work hard and stay positive. Lean on your family and friends, as we are here for you. We love ya. I'll be in touch and wanting to hear about your progress.

July 26, Tuesday, Email from Sammy P. (friend of yours)
Hi Susan.

I was just wondering if you could say hello to Trent for me. Everybody misses him and can't wait to see him again. I hope you're doing well out in Denver.

July 27, Wednesday, Email from Jo Ann (the mom of a high school friend of yours)
Susan, we were so sorry to hear about Trenton's accident. Chad

has not been in Kansas City this summer, but he received some information from Matt. I just talked to Rick last night and he filled me in on the details. Our thoughts and prayers go out to Trenton and all of your family. I know this is a devastating experience. Please keep us informed. We would like to send Trenton cards. Can you send us the address? I know Chad, Matt and some other guys would like to send a card too. We will all pray for the day you can bring Trenton home.

July 28, Thursday, Update from Me

Hi, I would like to thank Linda for keeping everyone informed regarding Trenton's updates. Thanks to so many of you, I can keep you informed with my new laptop. I appreciate this so much.

It has been somewhat of an adjustment for Trenton at Craig. It is a wonderful facility with a great staff. He is in a private room with a small living room area (my sleeping room) with a small refrigerator and microwave. In Springfield they kept him fairly sedated, which quite frankly Trenton liked, and here at Craig it is lots of work and they don't want him to sleep except at night, which he is having trouble doing. Once he is in more therapy classes during the day this should not be as big of a problem as he should be worn out at night. He has been fighting lots of stuff in his lungs which is suctioned quite a lot and bothers him and sometimes makes him sick, so he has not been the most comfortable. His spirits are somewhat down, but I think a lot of this is that he just does not feel that great. They will begin weaning him again in the next day or so and hopefully he will be able to start eating some soon. Progress is slow but it will happen. He is, as we all are, overwhelmed by everyone's generosity, love and support. He enjoys the cards he receives.

Please feel free to email me and I will continue to keep you all updated. Thanks again for everything. I don't think any of us could get through this without all of you!

July 28, Thursday continuation of my earlier update

Hi all,

My computer is acting up so I am on Rick's and trying to update you all so if I don't answer you individually it is because I don't have mine up and running right now.

It has been a good day for Trenton. He passed his swallow test, which means he can start having some real food. They will start slowly but it is exciting for him. Also, they have started weaning him from the ventilator. He has been off of it for 10 minutes today and they will up his time each day. They actually think this will go rather quickly, so hopefully he will be off in a week to 10 days. He sits in his chair for long periods of time, which is nice.

I am sorry this is pretty brief but I will write more when my computer is up and running. Also, they let him talk once yesterday and will again today.

So my computer . . .what a mess that was! My friends had bought me a laptop so I could work while I was in Colorado as well as provide updates, etc. Well, the computer wouldn't work; complete dud. I went to a Best Buy in Colorado and they told me the warranty had expired (I had it less than a week) and there was nothing they could do for me. As mentioned earlier, I am typically not someone who cries or gets hysterical in public, but nothing in the past month or so had been typical. Uncontrollable tears just started streaming out of me as well as a hysterical dialogue of what had been going on in the past 30 days. The manager was paged and I walked out with a computer that worked.

July 28, Thursday, Email exchanged between Jane and Me

I hope things go well today. I know it will be great having Rick there so you can take a break. Go out, have a good meal, go back to your room and try to relax.

We found out that we need to work through a charity to hold a golf tournament. Lindsay is talking to the Reeve Foundation about how to set this up. I guess most of the money would go there and then a percentage could be refunded to Trenton. Not sure. We may not have enough time to do the golf tournament, especially to do it well. I think it might be better to do it in the spring anyway when Trenton could be there.

I hope Trenton gets to feeling better SOON, for his sake and yours. I wonder if he caught a flu bug. I wish I would have just driven out with you. I feel like I should be there. I am still looking for a cheap, last-minute airfare. If you can just hang in there until Thursday you should be good to go until your return to take Jamie to school. PLEASE let me know if there is anything I can do from here. I can take the dogs again, or shop and/or cook for Jamie (and Ashley), etc. My heart breaks for what you are going through. Neither Nancy nor I are sleeping well these days either.

I know if it were one of my girls in Trenton's place, I would want to be there all the time too, but... you do need to give yourself long breaks on a daily basis. Trenton is in great hands and you need to make sure you are sleeping and eating to keep your strength up. And, take your medication!

My response to Jane

I don't know. No big deal. He had a little better night last night. He has a lot of congestion in his chest and they are suctioning tons. He has thrown up a few times also. Just scary for him. He is resting right now. Monday they will force him to get up and start therapy. They are letting him get by over the weekend.

I am fine. It is not easy, but will be fine. Once he is feeling better I will be better. Got quite a bit of sleep last night.

"I am fine" as my friends will tell you, is something I say quite a bit. It's not that I am fine, but there isn't much else to say. I have often argued that "fine" is a horrible adjective as it non-descriptive.

Y ou were not only feeling puny due to the effects of coming off the morphine, but also due to the fluid in your lungs. You learned very quickly that due to your injury you could not generate sufficient force to clear respiratory secretions. So basically, you couldn't cough. They do have an assistant cough for Quads, which is someone exerting gentle upward and inward pressure with both hands on the abdomen. This helps to produce a more forceful cough. To this day I don't think anyone has ever assisted you with a cough. You also couldn't vomit normally. Actually, it is quite scary to think of you vomiting, as aspirating would be very easy. You just don't have the use of those muscles to assist with coughing or vomiting.

July 30, Saturday, Email from Betty (longtime friend of mine)
How are both of you doing? Think of you guys often during the day. Is the regurgitate stage over with? Tell Trenton Hi! I wear my bracelet all the time........And I do believe in him; tell him to work hard. Stay Strong!

July 30, Saturday, John, who lived in Colorado, would send a few updates to your friends periodically.
I went by to see Trenton today and he is doing pretty well. They have started weaning him off of the respirator and will continue to do so for the next two weeks when he will hopefully be off of it for good. He went ten minutes this morning on his own and probably another ten minutes at least once this afternoon, if not twice. They will keep upping the time every day until he eventually needs it no more. The trach will probably stay in for a couple more weeks but he is able to start eating some more solid food. He can shrug his shoulders pretty easily but that's about it for now. He told me he can kind of feel his pecs. He also tells me that he's gonna be walking in six months. Not sure if it will be possible but at least he has high hopes and has a positive outlook. He wanted me to tell everybody hi and thanks for everything, I'm kind of relying on you guys to spread the word to anybody else that is interested. And if there are any e-mail addresses you can give me for anybody else, I will add them to the list. Let me know if there's anything you all want me to tell him when I go back this coming week.

Email from Stephanie (your hairdresser, who also raised money at her salon for a television for you)

Hi Susan, I would like to be added to your e-mail list to keep up with Trenton. You are both on my mind all of the time. I hope things are going well there. I'm sure it is a very difficult time. Please tell Trenton that I am sending my love and that all of my prayers are for him. Also, be sure to take care of yourself and know that many, many people are praying for you.

Love, Stephanie

Email from Nancy (high school friend of mine).

Susan, I just read your latest e-mail to the group. Susie forwarded it to me. I want you to know that our family has Trenton and all of you in our thoughts and prayers. We have a little bit of an idea what you are going through. I'll never forget Ashley bringing sandwiches to my son Brian's hospital room in Columbia. I was thrilled to hear that Trenton got to go to Craig. You couldn't have him in a better place. Mark's brother is the president of the KC Chapter of the Spinal Cord Society. He has been involved with this for around 17 years. All the fundraisers we do are for research to find a cure. He feels very strongly that it is just around the corner. If there is anything we can do, please let us know. I hope Trenton gets to feeling better. I'm sure that will help with a lot of things. I know the hospital staff will keep him busy. We will continue to keep all of you in our prayers. Again - if we can do anything, please let me know.

The following is an email from Matt Feeney who was an avid skier and mountain biker. In 1988 he was injured in a cliff diving accident at Lake Powell that paralyzed him from the waist down. He founded Adaptive Adventures.

Hi Susan. I wasn't sure if you saw the front page of the Rocky Mountain News today, but there was a great story about a friend of mine, Jason Regier, who is a quadriplegic and quite inspiring. I met Jason nine years ago at Craig Hospital after he was in a car accident. (He is a friend of Pete Ray, who I grew up with) Anyway, I thought you might want to see the story. I'm looking forward to meeting you and Trenton next week.

July 31, Sunday, Update from Me

Good morning. Trenton had somewhat of a restless night last night but otherwise is doing well. We took him for a little outing yesterday to get some fresh air. Since I am suction certified now, I can take him outside or around Craig. He does not like me to suction him because I don't do a very good job (his opinion), but in a pinch I would do.

They weaned him 20 minutes three times yesterday and I know he could have gone a lot longer. Today they will do at least 30 minutes. He hasn't eaten anything yet but I think the feeding tube makes him so full he just isn't hungry.

We have been filling him in on his drug-induced comments he made in Springfield and he is getting a kick out of that. His room is decorated with Chiefs stuff and the posters you all signed during the prayer service and the picture poster some of you made. He is ready to watch the tape of the prayer service, so we will do that today. I think this is progress, as before he didn't want to talk about any of this. His goal, as he will tell you, is to walk, and that is all he thinks about.

Last night at 4:00 am I heard the nurse tell him he was so polite and it was so nice to have a patient like that, even though he had called her about 20 times.

Jamie is coming in tomorrow and Rick and Cathy have been here this weekend. I will be here through next Sunday and go back and work a couple of weeks. Ashley, Tyson, Angela, Josh, and Lindsay are coming the weekend of the 19th to the 21st and I will be coming back after that. If you are planning a visit just let us know so we can coordinate. The weeks will start getting busy for him with classes but weekends they pretty much leave him alone.

Trenton sends his love and thanks for all your cards. The nurses always comment on what a big guy he is. I told them he used to be so skinny that he was Waldo one year for Halloween.

My email to Kay (longtime friend and Trenton's teacher in high school who only asked that Trenton come dressed to her first hour

class).

It is so nice to hear from you. Trenton got your letter yesterday and got quite a chuckle with you talking about Bill. He watched the video for the first time today of the prayer service and got pretty emotional, but smiled when you were telling your story. All in all, I think he is doing pretty well. Has been off the vent for 30 minutes today and wants to go longer tonight.

I am sorry I missed the party. Really wanted to go. I had heard it was so nice. Thanks again for thinking of us. It sure helps.

Email from Amy (neighbor and like another daughter to me).

Susan, I hope you and Trenton (and all of your family) have felt supportive arms around you over the last few weeks. Since I heard about Trenton's accident my church in Chicago (Bethany United Church of Christ) has included him in our weekly prayers.

I called Craig when I heard he was going to be transferred there. The woman answering the phones had been in an accident a few years ago and suffered a spinal cord injury. She seemed to gain so much from Craig that she now works there. I was so impressed with her and her spirit. I know Trenton will be in great hands.

Please keep me updated on his progress and give him our love. So many people are praying for him - I hope you feel the strength in Colorado.

Email from Alanna (mom of high school friends of yours)
Hello Susan,

Katie and Meggie have been friends with Trenton since grade school. I just wanted you to know that we are praying for Trenton and your family daily. There is not a day gone by that we haven't discussed Trenton, mostly about good times they've had with him. Katie and Nikki are best friends and she keeps us updated daily. Please know as a mother I feel for your pain. I can't imagine. Please know if love could heal, Trenton would be well. He is loved and respected by so many. Take care of yourself.

Email from Lexi (good friend of yours and at the lake with you when the accident occurred).

Hi Susan,

Thank you so much for keeping us all updated. I know that everyone here thinks about Trenton every day and continuously wonders how he is. I hope that you are doing well also. I am sure that everyone asks, but if we can do anything for you while you are not here, just let us know. Tessa and I would be happy to help. Please tell Trenton that I say Hi and that I miss him very much. Especially tell him that I can't wait to see him and I send my love.

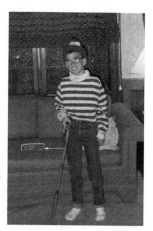

Email from Janine (good friend of mine).
Hi Susan,

I was just talking to Pat last night about you and the family, wondering how you were doing and if you were in Denver. I was just so upset when I heard the news about Trenton and wish I knew what I could do to help. Please, please know if there is anything you need or I can do for you, all you need to do is ask. As always I will keep all of you in my thoughts and prayers.

I am sure people have been sending you all kinds of research and info – so I am sure you have heard about the new documentary out called "Murderball." It is a group of guys who have been through what you are all going through now and how they have channeled their energy into this crazy wheelchair sport.

Let me know if there is anything I can send you or Trenton that will make your stay in Denver more pleasant. Be happy to send CDs or books on tape that he could listen too – just let me know. Also, please send on my thoughts to Rick as well. Not sure how to reach him.

Email from Trevor (good friend of yours).
Susan,

In case you were wondering who was sending you this e-mail, this is Trevor. First I wanted to thank you for having me on your e-mail list and keeping me up to date with how Trenton is doing.

I think about how he is doing daily and pray for him as well. But Trenton is strong, and always has been, which is what keeps me believing. I just wish that I could have been able to come down and see him before he was moved. I want him to know that he is in my prayers and thoughts.

This weekend was the benefit dinner for Frankie and I was talking to Gloria and the talk turned to how Trenton was doing. She asked me if I would send you her e-mail address to add to the list that you send out.

If you could tell Trenton that I am pulling for him, and that he is in my prayers, it would be great. I know that you are busy, but I did want to tell you that. So thank you for the time that you spend to keep all of us who cannot be there with him up-to-date. Thank you.

While you were in high school a good friend of yours was killed in a car accident. The benefit Trevor is referring to was for him. The tattoos you got were also in honor of Frankie.

Email from Vicki (good friend of mine).
Hi Susan. It's SO good to hear from you!

I can't tell you how much we have all appreciated Linda and now you sending out the Trenton updates. My family is rooting for, praying for and sending positive thoughts to Trenton, you and the whole family. Please tell Trenton that we all send our best!

Please let me know if there's anything that we can do here in KC to help you.............REALLY!

Email from Denise (one of my best friends and also going through her own nightmare).
Hey Susan,
Sounds like Craig Institute is just the right place. I went to their website and it looked really impressive. You must feel good knowing that you got Trenton just where he needs to be.

Remember to only worry about today. Don't think about tomorrow until you get up tomorrow morning. Telling a Mom like you and me to not worry is ridiculous but it has helped me to only think about the current day.

Brian has one radiation treatment left. We return to MD Anderson on Aug 15-16. They will do a MRI to look for residual tumor and we will go from there. Of course, our prayers are that the MRI is clear. The waiting is hell. In the meantime, he is enrolled at UMKC. He understands why but that doesn't make it any easier. Since he was little he was always Mizzou bound. I've tried to tell him this is just a curve in the road, but as you have probably found out, being too philosophical doesn't work. Take care and know that you and Trenton are in our constant thoughts and prayers.

As evident from the above email, friends were going through their own heartbreak. I truly was struggling with the "whys," and not, "Why me, but why anyone?" I still do.

Email from Mike (your cousin).

Thanks for keeping us updated. We really appreciate it because, as you know, all of you are in our thoughts every day. Again, tell Trenton that we said hello and ask if he has heard the Chiefs signed another cornerback. His name is Deyane Washington. He is a 12-year vet in the league. Tell Trenton that if he needs any updates on the Chiefs I would gladly give them to him because I listen to 810 all day at work to hear all of the news about the Chiefs.

August 1, Monday, Update from Me

Hi all,

Unfortunately this has not been a banner day for Trenton. He is running a pretty high temperature and feeling pretty bad all around. He was only up in his chair for about two hours today. No one seems too concerned about this. I have been trying to keep him awake so he might sleep tonight and he keeps cursing at me so I guess I won't wake him up anymore. The good news is Jamie is here so she is keeping me company, sort of. Laguna Beach is on so now I have no one to talk to.

I am looking forward to the Newfoundland dogs to come by. They do every Monday night and they are wonderful. There are six of them and they just come by to visit everyone. Mr. Grump told me they cannot come in the room tonight. Last Monday all six were in his room, which tells you how big his room is.

The respiratory therapist is in here for a wean session so I will write tomorrow.

Hopefully tomorrow will be a better day.

Of course I loved the dogs. They were so beautiful. Just seeing them made me smile. For some reason they annoyed the hell out of you. I was embarrassed to have to tell the kind man that walked around with them they couldn't come in. Oh well, I am sure you weren't the first patient that didn't like them (actually, I think you were).

Email from Ann (a friend we met through your dad's association with a trade organization called Builders Owners and Managers Association (BOMA).

Hi Susan,

Rick's been keeping me up to date on Trenton but I'd love to be added to your e-mail list to receive the updates. All the BOMA gang wants to keep up to date on his progress. Would it be okay to send something from BOMA?

Most important, how are you doing? Is there anything we can do for you - besides pray, which we're doing lots of?

Email from Sam (high school friend of yours).

Susan, This is Sam. I'd like to thank you for keeping us all updated about Trenton's condition. It means a lot to those who love him. Please wish him my best and tell him he is in my daily thoughts and prayers. I know he will meet his goals, if he sets his mind to it. Chris and Scott and I were talking about coming to Denver this weekend and I really wanted to know if you thought that was a good idea, Susan. Would Trenton even want us there so quickly, or would he like more time to adjust to his new environment? I'm wondering, because I don't want to upset him either way by coming when he is not ready for visitors or by not coming when he wants some company. What do you think?

P.S.-Do you need anything? Does he need anything?

Email from Lexi (a good friend of yours).

Good morning,

I just wanted to let you know that Tessa, Kristi, Derek and I are planning a weekend to come out and visit. We were thinking the weekend of September 16-19, but just wanted to run that by you and him first. We would love to make it sooner but with everyone's schedule it was hard to plan a weekend and we didn't want to bombard him with too many people at once. I will let you know for sure by Thursday the exact date, but just wanted him to know we are planning and WILL BE THERE. I hope that today is better for him. Tell him I miss and love him. Hope you have a good day too.

Email from Mary (the mother of a good friend of yours).

Hi Susan,

Sounds like a kind of rough day. I'm sure it's not easy for you and it goes without saying how tough it must be for Trenton. Are you able to go outside and walk around? What do the grounds look like? I can only imagine how hard it is - maybe you should make sure you get away by yourself a little each day to re-group.

Susan, you are doing a tremendous job just being there and being a mother. I guess in this kind of situation - the child, even though he is a grown man, reverts back to being the little boy that blames his mom for what goes wrong because they know you will love them no matter what.

I want you to know that I was talking with Marie over the weekend and, as you know, they have a fund of money they have collected over the years and Marie wants you to know they are more than willing to help you guys out with any expenses or with anything Trenton might need. You can contact Marie direct or let me know and I'll tell Marie.

What is happening about the stem cell treatments in China? Is that a possibility?

Do you have any idea how long Trenton will be in Colorado? Will the next step be to bring him home?

It's hard to believe that Jamie will be starting college soon. Gosh, I still think of her as being the cute little girl. Both of your girls have turned into beautiful young women. I know how proud you must be. I just talked to Kris, he is living in Oklahoma, and he said to be sure to tell you and Trenton "hi" and he is thinking of all your family.

Thanks for the updates.

Email from Gloria G. (provided the holy water and the mother of a good friend of yours).

Susan, I finally got your email address. I have been trying to get it since you guys got to Colorado. I want you and Trenton to know not a day goes by that we don't think about you guys and pray for you. I will be sending up some cards, now that I have the address, to the hospital. I just want him to know he is in our thoughts and in our hearts. Teressa hopes maybe with a little luck you will be back to bring him to the wedding. She really would like to have him there. Tell him to fight hard and we know things will go his way. Tell him we all send our love and can't wait till he comes home.

August 2, Tuesday, Update from Me

Well, Trenton is feeling much better today as far as no temperature. I talked to the nurse last night and asked her about this off and on temperature thing and she assured me it was very normal and not unusual for the first month to be one step forward and then two back. The problem I have now with him is he is very down and I don't know what to do for that. I know some of this will take time so I am trying not to get too concerned with this yet. He also won't eat, says he is not hungry, so they have cut back his tube feeding trying to get his appetite back, but so far no luck. We have a refrigerator full of apple juice because this is all he orders and then does not drink it.

The positive today is he was weaned for one hour at a time. He was not happy about it but he did it.

I again want to stress how much we appreciate all your emails, cards etc. They help us. I know he just has to work a lot of this out himself but it is difficult to see him so down.

I don't mean to sound negative. He really will be ok. A few of his friends are coming this weekend and I think it will do him some good.

Unfortunately, the good respiratory therapist has been off a few nights and we have this one who just ran over his tubing and he couldn't breathe for a few moments before she realized what she had done. So I better go and hope he makes it through this hour of weaning.

Y ou were definitely struggling. You didn't feel very well. Between the non-stop suctioning, temperature, coming off morphine and constant anxiety, I honestly don't know how you functioned at all. Of course, you were depressed. How could you not be? We all were. And yet the only thing we could do was to keep moving forward and take one day at a time. You really liked the staff at Craig. They were kind, but not overbearing and did not dwell on your injury. Yes, you were injured, but so was everyone at Craig. I tried to look around at the other patients at Craig and feel upbeat. I would often go outside, as most days it was absolutely gorgeous, and sit and watch people come and go. You know the saying, "It could always be worse." That was the problem; I didn't see a lot of the "worse." I saw paraplegics and wished so much you were just paralyzed from the waist down. One day during my trek around Craig I saw the patients with the brain injuries. I saw "worse" and was grateful you didn't have a brain injury as well.

Email from Cara (friend of yours)

Hi Susan, think about you every day. Trenton is lucky to have such a great mom standing by him...even if he sometimes gets fussy. Just thought you should know that I sort of giggled when I read today that Trenton has been saying "I'm not hungry" At the float trip/ fun in the sun/various gatherings when we were grilling out, Trenton ALWAYS starved himself...just cooks and cooks for everyone else but then never ate a thing. Same old Trenton . . . sheesh. I am forever grateful for your daily updates. It's great to feel like I am not in the dark, even if the news isn't the greatest all the time. I have faith in him; he is one strong guy...thanks to you :)

Let me know if there is anything you need, I'd be happy to do whatever I can out here in CA!

Email from Derek (your good friend who pulled you out of the pool and whose parents are keeping your dog, Willy for you).
Hi Susan, Hi Trenton.

First of all I just wanted to say thank you Susan for all the updates. I know you are busy and we all appreciate hearing from you every day. I also wanted to give Trenton a little update on how things are going here in K.C. Willie is doing awesome. He's being very good......well, he had one bad incident the other day and I had to put him in timeout! My dad baked a chicken and put it on the stove. Then before he knew it, Willie had reached up and snagged the chicken and started eating it on the floor. It was kind of funny. But other than that, he is well behaved.

I don't know if you've heard yet Trenton, but Scott and I were fishing the other day up at my uncle's pond and he caught a 7 pound bass! It was huge! We will have to send you the pictures. Sean is here and he just informed me that a couple of weeks ago Willie also snagged his sandwich when he wasn't looking! Jamie said she drove by and saw Willie outside and he's getting fat. So I guess we're feeding him well. Clarke says hi buddy! He has been at my house for days and I can't get rid of him. It's looking pretty good for Sean getting into the Police Academy in September. He has an interview in two weeks. This will be the last step for the process. Well, I have to go help clean the house. They're showing it here in an hour. We are all thinking about you and we miss you. I can't wait to see you buddy! Susan, if you need anything, don't hesitate to ask.

Email from Pat (a friend of mine).
Dear Susan, I guess you already know that Trenton's recovery is going to be filled with good days and bad.

You also know that it is the mom that has to be the strength that keeps everything going with a smile. I am not man-bashing....it is just the truth! Please know that Joe and I are thinking of Trenton and all of the family often...and praying for you all too. If there is anything you need or that we can do, don't hesitate to ask....I just don't know what to do to help. Is there anything we can do for Trenton other than cards right now?

My birthday, which was the last thing on my mind

Email from Lindsay (your cousin).

Hey Susan

Just wanted to say happy birthday! I hear you got some rest last night, which is good. I hope you get a chance to at least have a decent meal today or something. I'm glad Jamie is there to help you celebrate.

I just got out of a meeting with Michael and Tricia. They are the ones I've been working with in the Christopher Reeve foundation. They came by the office to see how Trenton was doing and to talk about what's been going on. They were very encouraging on the progress that Trenton will most likely make when he returns home. I know that Craig has told you that the feeling and sensations Trenton has when he leaves rehab will most likely be what remains. They said that is not true at all and that Chris gained the majority of his sensations he had after he came home from rehab. It is just a matter of how hard Trenton works at it. They are looking forward to helping out when the time comes so he can get the best out of what is available.

Please give Trenton my best. Michael and Tricia brought a couple books they wanted to give Trenton that I will bring out when I come. They talk about Trenton all the time in their meetings and wanted him to know they are thinking of him. Remember- there is that information center that the foundation provides for you if you have ANY questions on ANYTHING. This is a federally funded service that is designed to answer these types of questions. The lady's name is Bernadette and she is incredible. Please call her with anything. She will know who you are; I've spoken with her on several occasions.

HAPPY BIRTHDAY DARLIN!!! Tell Trenton I love him.

Email from Lisa (a friend from BOMA).

Dear Susan, Trent and family,

Henry forwarded an email updating Trent's condition and we were so glad to hear of his progress. You have been in our thoughts since the accident and we have been hearing bits and pieces of Trent's progress and move to Denver.

I wish there was something we could do to help. If there is any way we could support you all please let us know. Are you all staying at a hotel? Could we have the address there?

P.S.. I watch Laguna Beach too and can't believe the girls aren't in big trouble with their parents. They sound so insipid.

Email from Pam (college friend of mine).
Dear Susan, I was so sorry to hear about Trenton's accident, and have kept him in my prayers. I assume that you are in Colorado because it must have a special hospital for spinal cord injuries. Susan, I also pray for a cure and if it takes embryonic stem cells, then so be it (don't let my fellow Catholics know this is how I stand). I don't think they can understand until they are faced with a life-changing tragedy. My brother was diagnosed at age 31 with Lou Gehrig's disease (ALS), and we watched it take him in three years, where he had no quality of life. He left three young children. Embryonic stem cells could be used for a cure for ALS, Parkinson's, Alzheimer's and spinal cord.

How are you doing through all of this? Are you keeping a journal? I had a friend who made a website and kept his journal on it so that friends could be kept up to date. I don't know how hard that would be, but I'm sure there are many friends and relatives who are praying for him and anxious to hear about his progress.

Susan, all of us as parents are so fearful that we will get a call that says our child has been injured. Many never have to experience it. I pray that YOU are surviving this and keeping your faith and beautiful spirit. Denise told us that your birthday is Wednesday. Since you were a year behind me, would you be 49, or were you a YOUNG college freshman and this would be your 48th!? Do you know anyone in Colorado who is there to keep you company? I hope that in spite of all this, you can have a good birthday on Wednesday.

I'll be thinking of you that day. Please tell Trenton that there are people praying for him that he doesn't even know! God bless you all.

August 4, Thursday, Update from Me

Hi,

Well today was a very good day. I had a talk with him this morning and then the very good respiratory therapist had a very good talk with him also and what a difference! He was off the ventilator for an hour this morning before therapy and then after his therapy he was weaned again. At the hour mark he asked to go another hour so he was off the ventilator for a two- hour stretch. Tomorrow he has been told he will do three 2-hour weans. And Jamie and I got him to drink some of a milkshake and a few bites of chicken. He tried their cheesy potatoes and nearly gagged (a little dramatic) from the taste. His friend John, who lives here, came to visit for a few hours and he was very chatty. The nurse said he is her only patient who sits in their chair for such long periods of time. What a difference a day makes! I know we will have good and bad but I sure like these days better.

I also have to tell you that he gets more mail than any other patient, I think ever, thanks to all of you. It really makes his day and he is hearing from people he has never met, but I also want to explain why some of you get these updates twice. My email won't let me email to such a big group so I have to break it up and it gets confusing. It shouldn't be that confusing but it gets to be a long day.

Aug 4, Thursday, Update from John

I am sending this e-mail from Susan's computer in Trenton's room since I don't have internet access quite yet. When I got here he was doing his second wean of the day. He went for an hour the first time and then decided to combine his second and third into one 2 hour session. He is progressing very fast with his breathing and should be off of the ventilator in a week hopefully. The trach should come out at the same time; at least that's the plan. It will make it a lot easier for him to eat and do therapy without all the tubes, since they are restricting him from getting out of his chair for therapy. He just got done eating a little bit of dinner, and I mean a little bit. Only about three or four small bites of chicken and only one bite of cheesy potatoes, which he says are terrible. But that is more than he ate for lunch, so that's good. Tomorrow they are scheduling him for three shifts of two hour weans and he can go three hours if he feels up to it. He wanted me to tell everybody hi and he misses everyone and appreciates all of the cards and mail that he has received. That's about it for now; I will probably be back next week on Tuesday or Wednesday. I believe Scott, Sam, and Chris are coming out to visit this weekend and then Phil, Booth, and Shippee are going to be out next weekend. He seems to enjoy seeing people, so hopefully everyone can get a chance to make it out. If anybody needs a place to stay, let me know in advance and I'm sure it will be alright to stay at my place. We only have a two bedroom two bath but anyone is welcome. Gotta go but I'll keep you all updated.

Your life at Craig was fairly predictable. For the first few weeks while weaning from the ventilator you wanted someone to stay with you at night. You were still very anxious. I can't imagine what it must have been like and you really didn't want to talk about it. I loved staying in your room and was glad you wanted me there. As I mentioned, I didn't like my room. I felt so alone over there. I also didn't care if you kept me up, as you often did, because you required suctioning so much. Jamie was visiting one weekend and we literally fought over who got to stay with you. You finally told us we could both stay.

The first time you could talk and eat after the injury was exciting for us. I thought you would be eager to eat all of your favorite things. Instead you barely ate a bite or two. I didn't understand. Nothing sounded good to you. Courtney, one of your nurses, explained to me when you go without eating for so long, you lose the desire for food. I had never experienced this, but I was told eventually your appetite does come back, but it does take a while. It took you a few weeks to get any type of appetite back. It was actually kind of a problem. They were supplementing you through your G-tube, so then it was a balancing act between how much to supplement you so you weren't full and how much you would actually eat. Since your accident on June 26 you had lost at least 50 pounds. Granted, some of that you could afford to lose, but you were getting pretty skinny.

When you finally could talk it was bittersweet. Obviously, there were many days you didn't feel like talking and I didn't blame you. We watched a lot of TV. We started watching 24 with Keifer Sutherland. You said you were ready to watch the video made of the service at St. Charles right after your accident. I had not seen it either and was astonished how many people were at the church. The pews were full. There were readings and prayers and then it was left open for your friends, family and parents of your friends to come forward and talk about you. The stories were funny, heartwarming and heartbreaking. A lot of stories being told began with, "I remember when," as if you were in the past. At one point, Chuck said to the crowd, "Trenton isn't gone. He is still very much alive." It really didn't matter how the stories were being told; the fact that so many people came out to support you was amazing and I know you were touched beyond words. You were also fairly somber after seeing the tape. It was difficult for me to watch, so I knew it had to be hard on you.

At Craig, part of the process of rehabilitation is not only adapting to your new way of life physically, but emotionally. This involved going on "field trips" with other SCI patients. In doing so, we met and heard the stories of the other patients. All were equally touching as well as heartbreaking. I have never looked at life the same after hearing their stories. I think about them when changing a light bulb, seeing a car accident, hearing of someone going scuba diving. A SCI can happen from doing the most mundane activity to having a devastating accident.

Email from Brenda (who is a friend of your sister).

Susan, thank you SO much for all of the e-mails and updates. I have to tell you that I ANXIOUSLY await the update every evening. I am so happy that Trenton is doing so well. Brent and I are going to try to make it out there one weekend with Ashley and Tyson to visit him. I would love to see him and get to hang out for a few days. Please tell him and Jamie HELLO for me!

I am sure you have already heard this but Candace and Scott are going to have a baby GIRL! I am SO excited. I hope you and

Trenton have another great day tomorrow. Your family is always in my thoughts and prayers!! Have a nice night.

Email from Betty (a friend of mine).

Hi Susan. A belated Happy Birthday. I thought of you yesterday; just did not get to even read my e-mails. Keep your chin up with Trenton's attitude. Our chemo patients mentally go thru much the same depression and anger at their situation. I have seen this behavior many times before. Not that it is much consolation for you, but patients almost always strike out at their moms the most. It is that unconditional love thing. They are angry and frustrated and know that you will always love them no matter what. They feel safe in taking out their frustration on you. From what I have learned over the years they don't even realize they are doing it. Most of them really want to scream at the nurses, doctors, and anyone who is providing their care. They are just so sad and angry about what has happened to them. I think they are afraid if they strike out at anyone but family and the ones they LOVE the most, the strangers will no longer help them.

Don't be afraid to set limits with Trenton. Tell him you love him and want to support him, but need his love and support as well. From what I have observed over the years they are usually better with the fathers. Just like we all know, we can push our mothers a lot more, and have a little more fear of pushing Dad too far. Hope this helps make you feel a little better. Hope to see you while you are home.

Email from Joe (a good friend of yours).

Hi Susan,

It's Joe. Thank you for keeping me informed on Trenton's condition. Tell him hello for me. I am going to try my best to make a visit out to Colorado. Tell Trenton, when he gets back to KC we will try to get that beer gut back to rare form for him! Take care.

Email from Anthony (a neighbor and friend).

Dear Susan,

Please tell Trenton that I think of him daily. I always have his blue wrist band on. I wish there was something I could do for him. I have been praying daily for him. He is at the top of my list.

I sure hope that Philip and his friends make it there to see him. I am sure he will enjoy that.Give Trenton my best.

August 5, Friday, Update from Me

Hi all,

Today has been another good day for the ventilator weaning. He went two hours this morning before therapy and after therapy he started weaning again. We watched "Office Space" and then they came in to transfer him back on the vent and he asked to do two hours more. It took some convincing on Trenton's part, but they agreed. We watched "The Italian Job" so he was off the vent for a total of four hours this afternoon for a grand total of six hours today. Tomorrow he will do two 3- hour weans, just because that is all they can bump him up to. Sunday, he will probably either do two 4-hours stretches or six hours. They really expect him to be off the vent in seven days, which will help with so many things. He didn't eat anything today but we concentrated so much on weaning. He is still getting a feeding tube so he isn't starving. We just need to work on one thing at a time. Jamie left today, which was hard on all us.

When he goes to therapy they have his bed all changed and neat when he comes back, even though he stays in his chair until 10:00 pm or so. But today was so cute, as one of the nurses had taken the Royals bear Cathy had given him and laid it in bed with his call signal by the bear's lips and a towel over his stomach. That is how Trenton sleeps, with the call signal by his mouth so he can puff on it and a towel over his stomach because he is usually hot.

He has some great nurses, techs and respiratory therapists that are getting Trenton to smile and joke with them. They have been told not to come in his room without Ativan, which is an anti-anxiety medication. It is a big joke because Trenton is always saying he needs it when he is doing pretty well without it.

He is anxiously awaiting the arrival of Scott, Chris and Sam T. tonight. I hope I didn't ramble too much.

August 6, Saturday, Update from Me

Hi,

Trenton is sitting with Chris, Scott and Sam watching the football game. He is doing fine. Had a three hour wean this morning and will do another three hour one tonight at 6:30. Chris, Scott and Sam got in last night about 10:30, so they stayed until about 12:30 talking, which was great for Trenton.

He ordered a hot turkey sandwich and mashed potatoes for dinner, so we will see how much he eats.

I have to leave tomorrow morning so will rely on the nurses, as well as Rick when he is out here, to keep me informed for a couple of weeks so I can keep up with the updates.

They asked him his goal for this week. Apparently they do that, and he said to be off the ventilator, which is good. This next week he has more classes, so slowly he will start to be busy all day, which is good. I noticed he had a 9:00 class Monday morning. I feel sorry for whoever has him, as he is not a morning person.

August 7, Sunday, Update from Me

Hi all,

I left this morning around 8:00. Trenton ended up not doing another wean yesterday. He just was not feeling that well all day. Even with his friends he just did not feel all that great so he was not much company, although he was so glad to see them. I was very anxious leaving this morning but he had had a fairly good night. After the nurse, tech and everyone else assured me he would be ok this morning, I left. I called a few hours later and he was still sleeping and he had told the respiratory therapist he would wait to do a wean; I didn't like the sound of that. I called Courtney, his nurse tonight, and she said he was kind of down and had slept most of the day but had done one 3-hour wean and may try to do another tonight. It is so hard because you can't talk to him, and even though this might be good for him it is very difficult not being there.

Rick gets out there tomorrow night around 7:00 so he just has one day and he will have classes tomorrow, so he should be better. This is the first night he will have to sleep with no one in his room so I will have to double my doses of drugs to sleep tonight. (Again, somewhat kidding, but not entirely).

August 8, Monday, Email from Joe (a neighbor and friend of ours)

Susan, I know you and Rick have been deluged with messages. I wanted to send you a note with some information I think will be helpful. Pat and I get updates forwarded from Vicki. It goes without saying that Trenton is in our prayers.

I wanted to make sure you had a couple phone numbers I gave Lindsey but haven't heard if you or Rick had been able to use. I run an organization for physically disabled athletes (Mid-America Games for the Disabled). Steve Palermo is our honorary chairman and his wife, Debbie, is very helpful with getting us in touch with Steve's foundation for spinal cord injuries. I talked to Debbie when Trenton first got injured and she said Steve would very much like to talk to Trenton when Trenton is up to it. Having had Steve call the niece of one of my co-workers, I was told that talking to Steve was very helpful and uplifting for the young lady. Debbie also asked that you call her so she can talk to you about important issues. Debbie gave me their home phone number and asked (since it is unlisted) that you keep it confidential. Debbie's mother, Diane, runs their foundation and has a lot of helpful information you can use. Debbie is a wonderful woman and is waiting for your call.

I get the updates and know our prayers are helping, as it seems Trenton is doing better.

Email from Lindsay

Hey Susan-

Next Monday, the 15th, I am going to visit and tour the Stowers Institute in KC for work and would like you to come along. I'm not sure if you are familiar with Stowers, but they are one of the leading biomedical research organizations in the world. I asked Ashley a couple weeks ago and she is going to try to switch days for work so she can come along. I think you will find it interesting. They will be able to explain the impact of stem cell research and other research options they are pursuing in the field of spinal cord injuries. It is at 11:30 and would love it if you came along. Let me know if you think it's possible. Also, if there is anyone you want to come along as well, please feel free to invite them. Just let me know so I can give them a final number.

August 8, Monday, Update from Me

Hi,

Since I'm not with Trenton I don't have as much information, but I did call the nurse this morning and she said Trenton had his 9:00 am class this morning, which I said would not make him happy. He is not exactly a morning person. She also said his night went about the same as always. Rick got out there about 7:00 and Trenton had weaned for five hours, which is great, and he said he was doing pretty well. Rick joked with the nurse that he should just wean ten hours tomorrow and she said maybe they would let him wean seven, so we will see. He had received a lot of nice cards. The nurses always joke that they are going to start charging us per letter.

Touching emails from your friends

Email from Sam T. (a good friend of yours).
Susan, please read to Trenton
There is something I forgot to tell Trenton. It struck me on the long ride home from Denver that I forgot to tell him something, something that I wanted to say...So will you please tell him for me, Susan? Tell him that I said, "That he is gonna get through this..." I know that may sound rather naive coming from me or that it may not necessarily be my place to say, because I know Trenton is in a position right now where nobody who loves him or who he loves can possibly relate to him; but he is going to get through this. I know that in my heart and in my soul. It has always been my experience with Trenton that if he sets himself to something, that he will most likely accomplish it. After all, he is one of the most stubborn people I have ever come across. Besides myself.

Tell him, from me, that I like his odds. And that I believe when it's all said and done, that he will come out on the other side. God bless you Trenton. I love you. Don't know if I'll make it out there again. I may, but I'll be around when you get back to Kansas City. We'll sit down with a pack of smokes and I'll kick your ass at chess.

I was so touched by your friends who sent emails, cards etc. Their notes of concern and well wishes were heartfelt. I realized how devastating this had to be to all of them as well. While you were still in Springfield, Joel, a long time friend of yours, came by to see you. When he walked out, he was visibly shaken. I had friends tell me they didn't want to see you that way and some couldn't bring themselves to come to Springfield because it was too hard for them. I would think to myself, "But this isn't about you." Later I realized we all have different coping skills and, while not everyone showed their concern the same way, everyone did show their support.

August 10, Wednesday, Update from Me

Good morning,

I am resending this because I know some people were having trouble getting it. Sorry I didn't get this written last night, so here is for yesterday. Trenton can be a very stubborn and moody person. I know most of you are gasping because you had no idea. So the routine continues. They come in and say "Trenton, are you ready to wean?" And Trenton says "maybe later" and they walk out. A little frustrating, to say the least. So Rick had a little talk with him and the staff again, so we will see. He did wean for five hours yesterday but he could be doing so much more, which everyone agrees, so let's push him a little. But it is also important to remember (and I am saying this for my benefit) that of course he is going to get depressed and he has to work through this. I think all of us are so anxious (that word again) for him to get off the ventilator that we or I forget how hard this must be for him. All in all he had a good day yesterday.

Email from Cara (a friend of yours).

Hi Susan! My roommate in San Diego, Lindsey, has a brother who was in a motocross accident five months ago and is in a chair now. She is passionate on the subject, and inquires about Trenton's process so much that I have taken to reading her the daily updates you send :) She has a lot of faith in the community of people that her family has met through the tragedy, and would love to give you another shoulder to lean on. Lindsey's mom has even told me to "give Trenton's mom my cell phone number!" Ricky (her brother) has a fantastic attitude and seems very Trenton-like. His internet profile says, "Why walk when you can ride!" Haha!

Wasn't sure how interested you would be in speaking with her family, but I know they have done a lot of research and are very involved with the future of stem cell...thought I would bring it up to you, and then let you take it from there.:) Some pics of Lindsey and Ricky are attached for fun!

Email from Ryan (a college friend of yours).
Hello Susan,

My name is Ryan and I am a friend of Trenton's from Northwest. I would like to be on your forwarding email list so that I am updated on Trenton's progress. Thank you very much and tell Trenton that I am thinking about him and can't wait to see him when he gets back to KC.

Email from Matt (a high school friend of yours).
I just wanted to say that I've been reading every e-mail and enjoy hearing of Trenton's progress, especially days like Friday. My family, friends and I have all been thinking of Trenton on a regular basis, and wish the best for him. The size of Trenton's support group says a lot about him. He certainly has a lot of people praying. I hope things continue to go well. You're in our thoughts!

The weaning continues, as do the emails.

August 11, Thursday, Update from Me

Hello,

Today Trenton had a bone scan, as he has a calcium deposit on his hip and it could impede his progress, so now he will take medication for that. I was told this is not a big deal, and that it is fairly common and it can be treated. He was weaned for six hours straight today and Rick was not sure if they would increase it tomorrow or stay the same. Rick has also been suction certified and was attending a seminar on advancement in spinal cord research tonight at the suggestion of Dr. Chi (Trenton's doctor). They suggested since Trenton will not eat the hospital food that Rick offer McDonald's cheeseburger, etc. but he still did not eat today. Rick did want me to mention that the O'Dowd's event will be September 17th. I did call tonight and talked to Trenton and he clucks to let you know he heard you, so I am able to tell him things and update him on who I have talked to, etc. It doesn't sound like much, but it does help when you aren't there.

I forget what I have mentioned but if I haven't mentioned this, we do have his walls plastered with pictures that you send. For instance,

Trenton's grandma has sent him two pictures of her, and Nikki and Jackson are on the wall, as well as lots of his friends. So if you send a picture it will be on the wall. Rick and I also read him his mail and emails, so if there is a story you don't want us to know make sure you wait to share it with him when he does not need us to read it to him.

I am amazed at the contacts I have received through all of you and can't tell you how much it has helped. It is so nice to talk with those who have lived a similar situation.

I will hopefully tell you tomorrow he has eaten a Big Mac and weaned 12 hours.

Email from Patty (a friend of the family).

Susan:

Just to let you know that I have been reading all your emails and the ones from Ann Holwick since this terrible ordeal began for you and your family. They say that God never gives us more than we can handle, but boy, don't you just wonder sometimes what exactly He has in mind. Hang in there, your strength will definitely be what Trenton needs. Just know that there are lots of people out there cheering for all of you.

Email from Joni (a good friend of your Aunt Joni's)

Dear Susan, I wanted to let you know that I and my extended family have been praying for Trenton and your family too. Tim forwards me the e-mails as well as to my two sisters. It has been nice to keep up with his progress through Tim.

Just wanted to let you know that we are thinking of you often and praying for Trenton. What is the O'Dowd's event? Maybe we could attend.

Say hello to Rick and Trenton for me.

If there is anything I can do from here, please let me know.

Email from Teressa (a high school friend of yours)

It is so great to hear his progress! I love hearing from you every day, good or bad. It sounds like he is improving. As long as he improves a little bit at a time, I know he will be on his way to recovery. How long do they expect him to say in Colorado? When he leaves there will he come back to KC or will he go somewhere else for treatment? You probably do not even know the answer to those but I was just curious. What is Trenton's address there? I would love to send him some stuff.

Hang in there Susan. I know things will get better and, as always, I am keeping you and your whole family in my prayers.

Email from Sam's Uncle (Sam lived with you after you returned to Kansas City)

Susan,

This is an email from my uncle. The computer for Trenton is ready to go and is being shipped to my uncle today. It is not brand new, but they said it was put together so that it will run perfectly with the voice activation software that they use at the hospital (Dragon). As you can see they also put a DVD player in it for Trenton to watch movies.

I didn't know if Trenton already had a computer, but knowing how much he loves fantasy baseball and football, I thought this would be a way for him to continue doing the things he liked. Hopefully the hospital will start training him on the voice activation software. That way when he's ready to leave he'll already know how to use it.

My uncle and his co-workers have been working on getting a computer for several weeks. When we couldn't get one for you in time we decided that getting one for Trenton might be useful for when he leaves the hospital. My uncle and his coworkers have received every update you've sent out -- he says he gets people stopping by his office on a daily basis asking how Trenton is. He started forwarding your emails to coworkers about a month ago and now Trenton updates are the first thing they ask for every morning.

Anyways, just wanted to let you know the computer will be here at the beginning of next week. I'll email you when it gets in and I can drop it by to whoever is on their way out to Colorado next. Hopefully my uncle can still get the software donated, and he'll keep me updated on that.

So, tell Trenton that he needs to start scouting the NFL preseason games for fantasy football.

August 11, Thursday, 2nd Update from Me Today

I just talked to Trenton's nurse Courtney and she said Trenton was a little bummed, as his father had left tonight, and he gets a little down whenever someone leaves. But she had gotten him to eat a couple of bites of a sandwich and a couple of sips of a milkshake. When I talked to Rick earlier today Trenton was in Occupational Therapy, which is where he will learn to use devices he needs to function in life. For instance, his wheelchair has a blow puff device and he will eventually learn to do his own weight shifts by blowing or puffing into this and his wheelchair will either lean forward or lean backward so he is not in one position for too long, to help with skin issues, etc. As it is now, we have a timer and every 20 minutes we have to recline or incline his chair.

He will also be able to drive his wheelchair by the same method. He was not having much luck with this today as apparently he crashed his wheelchair into something. The big news and most exciting is he weaned for nine straight hours today, which is great. A few of you have emailed me with some messages for Trenton and some news and I forwarded that on to Courtney (his nurse) to tell him and I will also read those to him when I get out there. I have so many people to thank for various reasons, but mostly for just listening and keeping our spirits and hopes up. We honestly could not do this without you. I mentioned the O'Dowd's event on September 17th. This is a pre-opening party for the Trenton R. Baier Foundation. Rick will have the specifics, but I believe it will begin around 6 and go until midnight and everyone is welcome. Rick was really hoping that Trenton would be able to come. It does not seem likely, but I would not put anything past Rick or Trenton, for that matter.

If you have any questions about anything please feel free to email me.

So the therapy was a little disappointing to me. I understood you needing to learn how to drive your chair and we needed to learn how to transfer you in and out of the wheelchair with the Hoyer lift. We also worked on using a transfer board. We were taught how to get you down stairs and upstairs in your manual wheelchair you were in once, and that was in the airport the day you came home from Craig. It's been sitting in your basement ever since. I was frustrated. But I didn't know enough to know if this wasn't right. I was looking for the therapy where you might gain some functionality with your arms. Honestly, show any of us one time how to do something, watch us do it and we could do it. While I understood learning how to use all of your equipment was very important, I didn't understand why that seemed to be all we did. Of course there was stretching, etc. I was just hoping for more.

Email from Vicki (a friend of mine)
Hi Susan,

So good to hear that Trenton has made such great strides in the weaning process!

I just wanted to let you know that Anthony just this minute talked to Philip. The guys left for Colorado last night and spent the night someplace in Nebraska (they left from Maryville rather than KC). Anyway, Philip thinks they should get to Denver approximately 3:00 this afternoon.

August 12, Friday, Update from Me

Hi,

Unfortunately I don't have a lot of information tonight because the nurse was busy with Trenton and could not get to the phone. But thanks to Philip who is out there visiting, I do know that he weaned for 12 hours today. He said he was doing fine and in fairly good spirits. The nurse this morning put the phone up to Trenton's ear so I told him about the computer that Sam's uncle got him and also gave him several messages from all of you. He was doing a lot of clucking to let me know he heard me.

Have a great weekend.

Email from Tina

Hi Suzie, this is Tina, Ricky's mom. So sorry to hear of Trenton. I know these injuries won't last a lifetime. The advancements in medicine are so promising. There really is a lot of support out there. Please give me a call. I hope I can help in some way.

Email from Sammy P. (a friend of yours)

Hi Susan! I just wanted to thank you for keeping all of us updated every day. It really is nice to know when Trent is making progress and what his attitude is. I pray that he stays focused and optimistic (as hard as it may be at times) in order to rehabilitate as much as possible. I know that he can surpass all expectations. Also, I was just hoping that you could tell Trenton a couple of things for me. I still very much plan on coming out to see him in Denver, but I can't right now because I got a new job with Sen. Bond and have to move to St. Louis in a couple of weeks. Tell him that I would have loved to have driven out there with Shippee and Booth, except that, well, I would have had to be in a car with Shippee and Booth for many hours. He'll understand because he knows about Shippee's gas and about being around Booth for too long. (Hopefully he laughs at this). Also tell him that he was a great fraternity chaplain, He should know why, but if not, he used to let me and some others get away with murder, but would punish Chad like he was a pledge. Anyway, I'm excited to hear his reactions and happy (but not surprised) that he will have so many visitors out there. I cannot wait until everything settles down and I get to watch sports with him and make him do his goofy laugh that I miss.

Talk to you soon and thanks again.

Email from Casey (a college friend of yours)

Susan,

This is Casey, one of Trenton's friends from Northwest. I met you but am not sure if you remember me. I am here in Denver with Phil and Adam right now. I have been trying to get the emails forwarded to me from some people but that worked for the first few weeks and has somewhat stopped. I was wondering if you would be able to put me on the email list when you send out updates of

Trenton. I don't know if Jamie told you but I set up a website on College Facebook for Trenton and am trying to keep people updated through this site I created. If you could please put me on the list I would greatly appreciate it. All has been pretty good here in Denver thus far. I think we picked a good weekend to come down since you or Rick are not able to be here. We have been hanging out with Trenton for a few hours each day and he seems to like the company. We all have been joking around and watching ESPN or DVDs and just talking about old times and he seems to enjoy the stories and company. We are leaving here today but are sidetracked because he was asleep. We are going back in an hour or so when he wakes up.

August 14, Sunday, Email from Gloria G.(a friend of the family)

Susan, I been thinking about Trenton all weekend. Tell him that I have been thinking about him and said some prayers for him this weekend at church. Susan, tell him Teressa is honoring him in her wedding mass. Tell him we love him. Hope to talk to you soon. Let me know that you got back up there safe.

Email from Keri (sister of a friend of yours)

Susan-

I had a few questions about the Trenton R. Baier Foundation pre-party at O'Dowd's. Is it at the new one up North or is it the one on the Plaza? I was also searching on the web for something I could send Trenton that might help lift his spirits and I found this man that was in a similar situation as Trenton named Scott. It might be something that you want to check out. I read his bio and it was very inspiring. If there is anything I can send or do to lift his spirits just name it. It was encouraging to hear that he weaned for 9 hours yesterday. Trenton and your family are in our thoughts and prayers every day. I know that God is going to get Trenton and your family through this situation. The will and determination in Trenton's heart to walk again is more powerful and determining that any medical prognosis. I pray for his recovery every night. Thanks so much for keeping us informed daily. I look forward to every day hearing of Trenton's progress. Trenton and your family are in my family's thoughts and prayers. Keri

August 15, Monday, Update from Me

Hi,

I apologize for not getting an update out yesterday but Jamie left for MU today and I was busy giving her a sendoff. So I just got back from MU and talked to Philip and he, Adam and Casey are still with Trenton. Philip said Trenton was going for a 15-hour wean today, but they had put in a new trach and he was not feeling the best. I'm not sure why the new trach, but maybe the nurse can tell me tonight. He also said that Trenton had been in a pretty good mood most of the weekend. When I talked to the nurse last night she said Trenton was pink on his bottom and they told him to stay in bed all day. She said Trenton was like, "no problem." Any pink spot is just a start of a pressure ulcer and they just make sure they are not on that spot until it clears up. If they catch it early it does not take too long to clear up. It was great knowing that Philip, Casey and Adam were with him this weekend with Rick and me getting Jamie off to school. Philip would put the phone to Trenton's ear and I gave him several messages from all of you, plus, I am saving the emails and will read them to him when I get out there, which is the 22nd. Ashley, Tyson, Lindsay, Angela and Josh are going out Thursday and staying until the 22nd. I think Rick is going back out Tuesday so he is not often by himself.

We are hopefully getting the details about the O'Dowd's event soon and I will pass them on. It will be at the new one in Zona Rosa.

I think that is it for tonight. I do know he was not able to watch the Chiefs out there, which may have been a blessing.

During this time, your Dad and several others had been planning an event at O'Dowd's, a local restaurant and bar. The intent of the event was to thank everyone for their support, as well as to kick off the Trenton R. Baier Believe Foundation. You would not be able to be home in time for the event, but Tyson did film you so the tape would be playing during the event. You also spoke in the tape thanking everyone for all their well wishes and support.

August 16, Tuesday, Email from Nikki (a high school friend of yours)

Susan-

Hello! I just wanted to send you a little note to say hello and let you know I am always thinking of Trenton and you and Rick and Jamie and Ashley. You have about a million things running through your brain at all times and you still manage to let everyone know what is going on. That is amazing and it just shows what an awesome person you are and what a strong character you have. I am sure you hear this every day but we all know how strong Trenton is and while this is going to be by far the hardest thing he will ever have to face in his life, he will for sure make it through this okay and with your help and support he will be more than just okay. It is amazing to see the amount of people that care about and ask about Trenton on a daily basis. Everywhere I go I have someone ask me about him. I cannot even imagine what you go through.

Susan, while I have absolutely NO idea what you are feeling and what you are going through, I hope you know that I (and everyone else) am here to help you in any way I can. I would be more than happy to help out with anything regarding Trenton. I sent Chris Rau a bunch of addresses he needed for the O'Dowd's event but any other way I can help let me know. Also, when you are in town I would love to see you and hear all about Trenton and his progress and experience in Colorado. I am sure you are very busy but if you happen to get any free time please feel free to call or email me whenever. I also want to plan a long weekend to see Trenton fairly soon. Do you have any suggestions when would be best? I know Ashley, Tyson, Josh, Angela, and Lindsay will be there the 18th-22nd, but do you know what other weekends are already booked up?

Take care of yourself and please tell Trenton I said Hi and that I miss him and love him. Thank you for everything you do Susan!

Continuation of Nikki's email

I just wanted to mention one other thing. I just got done looking over the website you gave us, **www.missouricures.com,** and I think that coalition is amazing. It is great that you are taking on this whole issue of stem cell research so that we can all be more informed and educated on this very hot topic. I joined the coalition to stop the legislation banning somatic cell nuclear transfer and I think everyone else should do as much. Many people do not understand all that stem cell research can do for our medical community and for our society and you are right in thinking that they all have their own opinion but almost everyone needs to be more educated about it. Let me know anything else you find out about all this stuff as well. I am totally on your side and will do everything I can to help Trenton and your family in any way possible. Okay, I promise I am done now. I will stop bothering you!!

Love, Nikki

Somatic cell nuclear transfer is a laboratory strategy for creating a viable embryo from a body cell and an egg cell. The technique consists of taking an enucleated oocyte (egg cell) and implanting a donor nucleus from a somatic (body) cell. Dolly the Sheep became famous for being the first successful case of the reproductive cloning of a mammal. https://dx.doi.org/10.1089%2Fclo.2008.0041

August 16, Tuesday, Update from Me

Hello,

I have lots of information to give you tonight. I talked to Trenton's nurse Courtney and she said he was doing a 17 hour wean today. Obviously, he is sleeping through some of this, which is good, because a lot of times he gets nervous about going to sleep during a wean. It sounded to me like they would keep adding a couple of hours a day until he is able to get to 24 hours. Now I'm sure you are all wondering when he does 24 hours do they take him off the ventilator completely, because I am wondering the same thing. I think he then does several days and then they would consider him ventilator free. They will keep the trach in for quite a while after that, however, for several reasons. One is to make absolutely sure he is breathing ok on his own and I think he will still have secretions to suction. I know there are more reasons but I don't know them. I believe they will then put a cap on his trach so he will be able to talk. She said his mood was up and down but basically doing well. He is excited to have Ashley, Tyson, Josh, Angela and Lindsay out there this weekend.

*Today Ashley, Angela, Lindsay and I went to Stowers Institute and met with Sandra, who was wonderful, and had a tour of the institute. It is an amazing research institute. They have a website which is: **www.missouricures.com**, the Missouri Coalition for Lifesaving Cures. I understand everyone has their own opinion, but it is important to go to this website and understand the research they are doing. It is amazing and very informative.*

We also met tonight on the O'Dowd's event and more information will be going out in a "Save the Date" card. It is an event to thank all of you and the proceeds will cover the cost of the event. It will also be the kick off to the Trenton R. Baier Foundation, which will be to help spinal cord injuries. If you know of someone that would like to receive information and they are not receiving updates, please give me their email address and I will forward it on to Rick so he can get the information to them. Again, the date is September 17th. There will be food, drinks, band and an auction. Tyson is putting together a CD of Trenton. If you have a picture that you would like included to be shown to everyone (hint: a fairly clean one) in this CD please either send it to Tyson or mail it to him.

Well, you won't need a book tonight. Thanks for bearing with me.

Email from Frank (father of a high school friend of yours)

Susan, tell Trenton that I have and will record all of the Chiefs games on DVD for him to watch when he comes home. Tell him that we all miss him and that Michelle is on her way to San Diego for a job. Tell him not to worry about her; two guys are driving the girls out so that they can all rotate the driving.

Email from me to Diana, a high school friend in Las Vegas

(I don't even remember having a going away party for Jamie)
Hi Diana,
I just got back from taking Jamie to MU. I had a party last night

for her. Of course, it was raining so I put tables up in my garage as I had about 30 people. It went well. Just family and friends.

No, the potty training did not go that well. They don't seem to be trained yet. I am just so tired to even mess with it. Ric 2 will hopefully try to get it done.

How is everything else? I am getting ready to send out an update. Didn't have time last night.

Diana's response

Holy Cow, Susan! I knew you were getting Jamie ready for MU, but I can't believe you had a party for her too. You have gone beyond the Supermom award. I don't know how you did that with everything else going on. You must be ready to drop from exhaustion - mentally and physically. But I'm sure you enjoyed an evening of fun surrounded by family and friends, even though it was a lot of work for you.

How does your schedule look the rest of the week until you go back to Denver? Will you have any down time to relax? If Ric 2 is willing, let him handle the girls for a while. That's one thing you wouldn't have to worry about then. Is there anything else you can delegate to someone else? You know you have a lot of people wanting to help you. Let them do just that, even if it seems like a little thing to you.

I'm sure it's hard being away from Trenton right now and with Jamie gone. Hang in there.

Take care of yourself. Don't feel that you have to write right away . . .

The girls Diana was referring to were my two puppies I mentioned earlier. Ric 2 and I had gotten them two months prior to your accident. As I said, they weren't trained yet and very stubborn about it. I actually ended up taking them to a woman who kept them and worked with them for several weeks. Potty training was the last thing on my mind.

August 16, Wednesday, Email from Ryan (a friend of yours)

What's up Trenton? I have been receiving all the emails from your mom and it sounds like you are doing a great job with your breathing. Keep up the good work so that you can come back to KC soon.

Kristy, Swank, and I moved into a condo off of 35 South and Lamar. We all think we are high rollers living there. Swank started teaching 1st grade this week so you can only imagine him running around with all those little kids. Kristy is starting nursing school at KU Med and I will be starting my 2nd year of PT school at KU Med. I am looking forward to hanging out again and definitely watching some Chiefs games. I really think that this is our year to win (although I do say that every year).

So are there any good looking nurses? Talk to you soon.

Email from Ann (friend of ours from BOMA)

Susan.

Thanks for keeping me up to date each day on Trenton. I'm forwarding your wonderful e-mails to many of your friends around BOMA who want to be kept up to date. It sounds like he's making great progress on the weaning and that his moods are a little better. I know that makes it easier for everyone around him. It's great he's getting all the good company to help lift his spirits. Could I please get more information on the new foundation you're starting in Trenton's name? Word has gotten around BOMA and I'm getting questions, so if you can give me information I can circulate, I would appreciate it. BOMA's Winter Business Meeting is in Tucson next January 13-18th. I know that's a long time off but you might want to give some thought to attending. You may be ready for a long weekend away by that time. Something to think about…..

Email from Casey (friend of yours)

Susan

I don't know if this is my business to ask or anything like that but I was wondering something. I remember Trenton's grandfather passing a couple years ago and I remember Trenton taking it pretty hard but there was one thing that seemed to ease his mind about it.

I remember him keeping his grandfather's candle and I remember Trenton being very proud of it. If you don't know which one I am speaking of my best description is a standing white candle with a picture of his grandfather and a paragraph all on top of an American flag. I was wondering if you might want to bring it maybe to ease his mind just by having it close to him. I was just wondering because I didn't see it and he always kept it near. I just wanted to tell you that and for you to do whatever you feel would be best for him. I apologize if this is none of my business to ask or speak of but it was just something I noticed for the last two years and just thought I would have seen it there. This is just something I thought of while I was visiting. On another note I did in fact receive the emails that you have sent since you put me on the list. I am also sending a few pictures and a card sometime in the next week or so and something I want to give Trenton. Maybe you will be able to read it to him when he gets there or whoever is there can do so.

Thank you and again, sorry if this was none of my business. I meant no disrespect. I just thought he might like to have it there.

I was so impressed with Casey for thinking of this. I knew exactly what candle he was referring to and we did get it and bring it out to Colorado. You were very close to Delmer and Casey was right. You would want it near you.

Email from Nathan (who was a fraternity brother of yours)
Hi,

My name is Nathan, one of Trenton's fraternity brothers. I have been talking with Lindsay about events and philanthropy stuff to do in Maryville and she has been forwarding all your emails to me so I can forward it to everyone in the fraternity.

If you could give my email address to whoever needs it so that I can get information about the Trenton Foundation that would be great. Sig Ep is going to make it a part of our philanthropy, alongside the Christopher Reeve Foundation. We are planning a lot of events right now and any info about Trenton's foundation could help us out greatly.

Please give Trenton my best and that we are all thinking about him. Also, I just got my wisdom teeth out today and so if this doesn't look too professional and some words are misspelled, I apologize. Oh yeah, I almost forgot, I work on Staley Farms Golf Course in Kansas City. I have worked there for the past four summers. I have talked to some people about what kind of help they could offer in regards to the golf tournament you all are planning or in just some sort of donations. They informed me that Staley Farms Golf Course loves to do that sort of stuff and that if I ever needed help with anything or the foundations needed help with anything to let them know and they could figure something out. Let me know what kind of help is needed; volunteers for anything.

Email from Jeri (a neighbor of ours and her children went to the same babysitter when you were growing up)
Dearest Susan,

On behalf of my family, I wanted to express our sadness on hearing about Trenton. You, Rick, Trenton, Ashley and Jamie have been in our thoughts daily since we heard from Sandy. I just wanted to let you know that you will continue to be in our thoughts and prayers for days to come. We are very interested in Trenton's progress! Sandy is good to forward some of your emails so that we know how everybody is doing. We've watched him grow up, as with your girls, and realize that you have some battles ahead. But also know that we all are lifting you up in thought and prayer right now. If you feel like adding us to your distribution list, that would be wonderful. If you need anything other than our support, please call upon us.

You are nearly vent free

August 17, Wednesday, Update from Me

Hi,

Trenton went 19 hours off the ventilator today and will go 24 tomorrow, which is so exciting. If he goes 24 hours for three straight days he is considered weaned. They will still keep the trach in indefinitely until they are sure no more surgeries etc., but they will do a balloon deflation device so he can talk. I forgot to ask if he was eating because I was so excited about the weaning so he may be skinny but he is breathing on his own. One thing at a time.

Also, the O'Dowd's date had to be changed. I believe it will be September 22nd but will let you know for sure. I also don't have a lot of details about the foundation, as we need a professional to set this up correctly. Can you tell I am tired tonight? Can't think. Anyway, I apologize about the O'Dowd's event. And as soon as I have the details for the foundation I will let you know how it will be set up.

Email from Sean (a college buddy of yours)

Susan-

It's Sean Dugan, one of Trenton's old roommates from college during 03-04. I've been getting your updates from Becky Crane and I read the recent one in which you mentioned something about the Stowers Institute. I just started at American Century and the Stowers Institute is one of the owners of American Century. If there is anything I can do please let me know. I know I'm only one of the "little guys" there and just started but if I can try to do something I will. Also, can I please be added to your list so Becky doesn't have to keep forwarding me the updates? And please tell Trenton I am thinking about him and hopefully will be able to make it out to Denver sometime soon. Thanks a lot!

Email from Diane (a friend of mine)

I have been wanting to email you for a while now. I have been praying for Trenton and your family. Julie forwards me your updates.

Trenton is really progressing well with the ventilator weaning. I know that must seem like a very slow process to you, but he continues to move forward. Sounds like you are learning a lot about health care and all people and processes involved - which I know can be overwhelming at times. I have to say that you are doing a great job with Trenton - he is so lucky to have you for his mom. Please know that I am here for you if you need ANYTHING. Hope to talk with you soon.

Email from Caitlin
Hello,

My name is Caitlin and my sister and I are friends of Trenton's and if you could add me on the email update list I would appreciate it. I know you are pretty busy so just whenever you get a chance. I have someone forwarding me the emails right now, but I would like one of those "save the date" cards. If you could tell Trenton that Carlie and Caitlin, "the twins," are thinking about him that would be great. Thank you.

Email from Chyleen from Iowa (a cousin of your grandmother's)
Dear Susan,

My mother, Evelyn, is a first cousin to Joan. I am the closest daughter to Wes and Rick's age. We spent many Sunday dinners picking on each other as kids. You and I have never met, but I am in KCK now and have been for a little over a year. My sisters are Lavon and Shirley, and I have a brother Gerald. We recently sent a card to Trenton.

Please know that we have you, Trenton, and your entire family in our prayers daily, as well as the prayer chain at my church in Bonner Springs, KS. You must be one of the best mothers in the world. I don't know how you can do all that you are. Strong faith will get you through this.

If there is anything our family can do to help you, please let us know. Please share this with Rick. I am very disappointed that on the day of the benefit my husband and I will be leaving for San Francisco and will have to miss the event. I would appreciate being kept posted, just in case. I would like to donate something for the auction. I don't have any on hand at the time, but I think I can get a nice baby quilt made. Would that be acceptable?

My mother Evelyn is not doing well in Fontanelle Nursing Home, and I have a close cousin on the other side of the family that is dying soon in Michigan, but I can certainly get a quilt of some kind made, either baby or adult.

Dear Tim has been so wonderful to keep us informed and has put us on his contact list, so we get your emails daily. I forward them to my two sisters. We are grateful for this connection.

Email from Karen (a friend of mine)

Susan, due to mutual friends and acquaintances I have been updated on what is going on in your life. I am so sorry for the unexpected turn of events and I know the life that you knew before has been changed forever. I understand that Trenton is now in Colorado at the Craig Hospital. What is the prognosis in regard to Trenton's ability to move, breathe, etc.? How is Rick B. doing with all of this? It feels like a long time since I have seen you; I hope you are holding up okay. I was very sad to hear about your son's accident. He is very lucky to have a great Mom to help him through this.

It was nice for people to think I was doing a good job. I don't know what else you do. If I am being honest, most days I didn't think I had it in me to even get up. Even now sometimes I think you think I am feeling sorry for myself. Maybe you don't understand unless you are a parent. My grief was and is seeing you sad or hurting. I just wanted, and still do want, to take away your pain. You do what you can knowing it isn't enough. I would pray for me to be in that bed and you looking over me. I wasn't doing anything any other parent wouldn't do.

You did it! Vent free!

August 18, Thursday, Update from Me

Hello,

I just got off the phone with Rick and Trenton will be completely off the vent by Monday if all goes well, which it looks like it will. He is busy in his therapy classes learning to drive his wheelchair and do weight shifts. He wants to concentrate on getting off the vent and then he said he would start working on eating. Right now Tessa and Derek are out there with him, as well as Rick, so I think he is in a pretty good mood. I gave Ashley quite a few pictures to take out with them tomorrow.

All I can tell you about the O'Dowd's event is that it will be September 22nd, which is a Thursday night. Rick and Cathy are planning the event and questions should really be directed to them. I would suggest contacting Cathy at CB Richard Ellis. The main number is xxxxx and ask for Cathy. I believe there will be information sent out soon. I will make sure all of you are contacted but if you know of someone who is not on my list please give Cathy a call. Thanks again. I love hearing from all of you.

Email from Judy (a BOMA friend of ours)

Susan - I just wanted to let you know how sorry Dick and I are about Trenton's accident, and also to send our thoughts and prayers to you and the family. We have shared a lot about our kids, particularly Jeff and Trenton, over the years and I can only imagine how awful this must have been (and still is) for you. We occasionally get updates on Trenton from BOMA and I am very much interested in his progress and pray for his continued recovery.

I hope you can all stay strong and keep faith. We will continue our prayers on this end.

Email from Chuck (high school buddy of yours)

Susan,

My cousin Kristi and I were going to fly out to see Trenton

sometime in September. Is there any weekend that is better than others? Tell Trenton I am anxious to see him, and I think about him every day. I also wanted to tell him that we are paying Trenton's entry in our annual fantasy football draft, which will be at the beginning of September. I know he will be excited about this, beings the fact that we used to talk to each other after just about every play. I have to get back to work, and thanks for the updates.

T.... Stay Strong

Love you man, see you soon.

August 19, Friday, Update from Me

Hi all,

I know this update is a little early but I thought it was important to tell you that I just heard from Rick and they (Craig) have decided to pull Trenton off the vent today vs. waiting until Monday. I asked Rick if he was nervous and he said, no not at all. Ashley and Tyson are taking their web cam so tonight I will be able to see Trenton hose-free. Unless there is more fabulous news like he ate a pizza tonight, I probably will wait until tomorrow for the next update.

Email from Ann (a neighbor and friend).

Hi,

You and your family have been in our thoughts and prayers every day since I heard about the accident. I have been getting updates from anyone I see that I think would know some news. I was happy to hear from Vicki about the emails. I know Bob thought getting out info when I was sick was wonderful via emails instead of all the phone calls. It is wonderful having all the support but all the calls can be exhausting. Please let me know if there is anything I can do. Robbie is living up in Milwaukee temporarily but wanted Trenton's address. Is there anything he enjoys from the guys? Anything that helps on a bad day? I told Robbie I got the address from Vicki and he should try and think of some funny little dumb things to write that Trenton might get a chuckle out of.

You seemed worried about his eating, which I can understand. I always hated cranberry juice but when I got back on food I loved it. I found anything with a strong flavor was sooo good. I craved

Mexican and pizza. I know you are getting a lot of good advice so I'm sorry to throw more out there.

If you wouldn't mind, please add me to your email list.

Email from Stephanie (your hairdresser)
Hi Susan.

Sorry I haven't touched base for a while. I am so happy that Trenton got off the vent. That is excellent news, he should be very proud of himself. Please tell him that I said "good job." So the total on the wristbands is now over $2100. I really do want to try to get out there to see him. In fact, I am hoping to try to talk Nancy into coming with me, maybe Julie too. We'll just have to try to figure out a good time. How long will he be there? Do you know yet? I'm so glad that he has had so much company. He really does have some wonderful friends. I guess because he is so wonderful! My brother and his wife had a baby girl Tuesday morning so I am leaving today to go see them in St. Louis. I will be back Monday and will try to talk to Nancy to see if we can get a plan together. Please give Trenton my love when you get back out there. Have a safe trip, and like always, take care of yourself. You all are always in my thoughts.

After your accident, Stephanie had started selling your Believe bracelets at her salon. She made quite a bit of money and with that money she bought you a flat screen television.

Email from Nathan (fraternity brother of yours)
Hi,

Well, I got some awesome news. I have been talking to the band, The Sound and The Fury, and the Sig Eps have got them to come up for a benefit concert in Trenton's name on October 14th, a Friday. The band has been getting bigger and bigger the past couple of years. They have played at 98.9 The Rocks, Rock Fest in Kansas City and also have opened for the huge band Chevell. The Rock plays their music regularly now in Kansas City and I had a chance to see them in concert last year and they are awesome. The concert will be raising money for the new foundation for Trenton that you all have been telling me about, as well as money for the Christopher Reeve Foundation. Another reason this is huge is that it is the weekend before homecoming. So we will use this to help publicize and have a start off for our teeter-totter-athon the following week. No contracts have been signed yet but they are in the mail and on their way. I will be talking to the venue guy this coming week in Maryville to get it all ironed out. I will let you all know the specifics when it becomes solidified. The band's website is **www.thesoundandthefury.com**. Clicking on the "psycho fans" part, I think, leads you to some of their music you can hear on the internet. I can't even begin tell you all how pumped we are to get this big of a band up in Maryville for the benefit concert. The radio station on campus is going to help us promote it. We got the venue for free; the band is only charging us $250.00 (plus the shelter, food, and beer) and now we are getting free publicity on the radio. So far everything is coming together to make this an amazing event. I will keep you all informed about the details when more come in.

Nathan was a fraternity brother of yours. He reached out to me regarding hosting a fund raiser at NWMSU. He also became quite involved in stem cell research. I got to know Nathan and was so impressed with him. The event was a Friday night and Nathan had a band and had asked me to speak. I am not much of a speaker, but I found that when you are speaking about someone you love so much, the fear of speaking lessens. I think I did all right and the event was a success.

August 20, Saturday, Update from Me

Hi,

Trenton is doing great being off the vent. He also has his cap on his trach so he is able to talk. It takes some time to get used to and it isn't real fluid but it is wonderful to hear him say anything. All he said to me was "yes" to, "Does it seem weird?" and "no" to, "Do you need me to bring anything when I come out?" and, "thank you" to me saying, "I am so proud of you for getting off the vent," but it seemed like so much more. When I get out there on Monday you can call me on my cell if you would like to talk to him. I decided to drive, as I will be out there for two weeks so I won't get there until 5 or 6 pm. Ashley also said that they were giving him more of the appetite stimulator so that hopefully he will start eating. Also, after Trenton went off the vent yesterday afternoon Rick called the gal who cuts hair for the hospital and she came over and shaved Rick's beard and also trimmed up Trenton's hair. He is waiting for you, Stephanie, for his real haircut. Kind of a big week.

P.S. Ok, sorry, but I made a big boo-boo. Ashley read my email and called me saying that he is only able to speak for three 10-minute time slots a day and it wears him out as he sort of has to burp as he does it, which you would think would be a piece of cake for Trenton, but anyway, they will slowly increase those time slots each day but it may be a bit premature to have you call Monday night. But I can assure you when he can talk to you I will let you know. I am so sorry for this wrong information.

Your father had not shaved since your accident, with the intent that he would shave when you got off the vent. I am pretty sure everyone was excited about this as well, since your father was not meant to wear a beard!

Now you're talking

Nothing is quick or simple with a SCI. I assumed, again stupidly, you would be vent free and just start talking away. You know, just like when you could finally eat; I thought you would eat everything in sight. Everything is a very slow process and takes time. Patience was not my strong suit and I knew it wasn't yours either. But, I had to keep in mind you had not spoken a word since June 26 and it was now August 19; nearly two months later. But the good news was you could talk and I didn't care how long at a time.

August 21, Saturday, Update from Me

Hello,

This has been such a great weekend for the kids to be out there. Trenton has been in a good mood and Ashley fixes his hair each morning. Lindsay stayed with him last night and Ashley and Tyson the night before. Ashley said Trenton had his Derrick Thomas jersey and she had the Trent Green jersey on, so they took pictures. Then Bridgett (his nurse) came in with a Broncos jersey. I was able to talk to him a little longer today. I think he was going for an hour with the cuff deflation so I'm sure he talked to Rick and Jamie and Chris and then last night he talked to his Grandma Joan. Ashley said it was probably a good thing that I am driving out because he is not eating the hospital food but is asking for Wendy's chicken fingers. Then they were going to take him out to the patio to eat. (Ashley is also suction certified, as of last night). I can't believe how far he has come in the two weeks I haven't seen him. When I left him that morning I made him promise he would work hard and not get too down. He promised he would work hard but said he couldn't promise the other. I think he has done both and a lot of that has to do with the support he has gotten from all of you. The cards, pictures and emails keep him going and wanting to reach his goal.

August 23, Monday, Update from Me

Hi,

What a difference two weeks makes! I walked in about 5:00 and he looks great. He is able to talk for 12 hour stretches and is doing really well but it does make him tired. He is eating better. He has had small amounts of pizza, chicken nuggets and milkshakes. He told the staff he was tired of messing around with his wheelchair (learning to drive it, etc.) and to start working him in physical therapy. Trenton really enjoyed the visit with Ashley, Tyson, Angela, Josh and Lindsay and was happy with the way they decorated his room with all the pictures, etc. He wanted me to thank you all for the pics, CDs, cards and all your support. I can't believe what he just did. I am working on this email and I hear him say no thanks, and it was to the guy with the Newfoundland dogs so I missed them. I am kicked out of the apartment tomorrow so I will be spending the day moving, I'm not sure where, but I will write tomorrow.

Email from Deidre and family (friends of the family)

Hi, Susan.

I look forward to your updates on Trenton each day. I forward them to Michael. Tell Trenton "hello" from Deidre and family. I believe you said Rick is taking the lead on the O'Dowd's event to kick off the establishment of Trenton's foundation. Can you re-send me his address/email? I told Janet about O'Dowd's and how I thought it would be nice for Winnetonka (especially the soccer program) to participate. She hustled right down to Mark's office. I told them I'd get the latest dates and times and get back to them. Take care of everyone out there--and that means you too! Deidre

Email from Vinnie (a friend of ours)

Susan,

Know that my family's thoughts and prayers are with you at this time. We are thinking very positive thoughts and I hope only for the best for you and your son.

Email from Sally (a friend of mine)

Susan,

Shanna is getting a poster signed by ALL (or as many as she can get) the KC Chiefs cheerleaders. Don't tell Trenton until we get it done. We will surprise him. It was good to see you last week. Remember I have an extra bedroom that is quiet or you can just come over and lie on the sofa while I am at work if you need some time to yourself. Have a good week. Sally

PS. I am sending this from Barry's office because lightning put out my modem at home. That was all, thank goodness.

Email from Debbie (your cousins wife's mother)
Hi, Susan,

I'm Debbie, Lisa's mom. We met at Mike's graduation. Nancy has been sharing your wonderful updates about Trenton with me, and I wanted to contact you directly and thank you for sending them. Also, I want to tell you how much I admire your strength, courage, faith, and positive outlook. Please know how much we all appreciate you, and how much we pray for Trenton and for your family. The progress he is making is awesome, and I'm certain he will continue to make great progress! Please let us know what we can do. I look forward to meeting Trenton when he returns from Colorado. I feel like I already know him.

I'm sorry that my husband, Dave, my daughter, Rita, and I will be in California the 22nd of Sept., and will miss the event at O'Dowd's. Rita's husband is returning from Iraq the end of September and we are flying out there to help Rita get settled. Hopefully we'll get to see Dakotah, but since the US Marines don't give an exact return date, all we can do for sure is get her out there, and then we'll come on back and she will wait for him. They will both be back here for Lisa and Mike's wedding.

Thanks again for the updates. I just wanted you to know I appreciate receiving them, and I appreciate you taking the time to send them. I know it is a comfort to your family, and the rest of us find comfort in them also.

Email from Sammy .
Hi Suzanne, (although I usually go by Susan, I also can go by Susie, Suzy, etc.) I'm glad to hear that you're doing good and going back out to be with Trenton. Could you please let him know that

I'm extremely excited (but again, not surprised) that Trenton is working so hard and off the trach. But I am surprised that he wants his hair styled every day. I hope he's not becoming a metrosexual like Quisenberry (ha ha). Actually, I don't blame him for wanting the only three hairs left on his head styled (ha ha). Anyway, the good news has made my day. I hope to hear more soon and will hopefully get to see Trent on the 22nd. I will definitely be making the trip home from St. Louis either way. Knowing him, he will probably be the hardest worker, as well as nicest guy, that the staff has ever seen out there. I can't wait until I can call him on your phone, but until then, I hope to hear from you via email.

Email from Allison

Hi Susan, I just got to work and checked my daily email about Trenton as I always do. I am so happy that he is getting to enjoy his company while they are there and that he will definitely be ready to see you when you get there. It's also great to hear that he is actually craving some kind of food! A lot of good has happened to him since you have been in KC. I bet that makes you that much more anxious to see him. I am always trying to think of things to send him, pictures, etc....but I can never think of anything, so if you have any ideas please let me know. I'm glad that he is making progress. I hope this continues because I'm sure it keeps his spirits high. Tell Trenton that I'm smiling after reading your email about his progress today because it is so good to hear that he is enjoying his company and sounding like himself. I know this great progress will surely be continued.

On another note, I bet you are relieved all this rush stuff is over with Jamie. My sister said she wanted Alpha Delta Pi and I knew she would get it. Now they can enjoy that, and then try to concentrate on school!

I hope your drive to Colorado is a safe one, and I'm sure Trenton will be glad to see you. I'm still continuing the prayers and thoughts for Trenton and all of you.

Email from Adam (a friend of yours since grade school)

I was wanting to know if I can get Trenton's address in Colorado so I can send him some things. What do you think I should send? What does he want? I have a DVD burner and can burn him DVDs if he wants. I have a huge list of DVDs so if he wants to choose I can send him what he wants. I have the new Sin City movie; ask if he has seen that, if not I can burn it and mail it to him.

August 24, Tuesday, Update from Me

Hello,

I have to give Trenton so much credit. He has helped me this time. I won't say that he is always upbeat but he really is pretty amazing. They worked him harder today in physical therapy because he wanted them to and he can do his own weight shifts if forced to and without too much cursing. He is able to talk for more than 14 hours, although he obviously doesn't talk the entire time and it does wear him out. He ate two chicken nuggets and about a 1/4 of a chocolate shake. He has won over all the nurses and techs. Today Courtney hit his foot pretty hard when moving him and I asked him if it hurt his foot and he said "Mom, I can't feel my foot, remember." We just finished Coach Carter and now they are getting him ready for a shower. Yesterday he was talking to Jamie and telling her to make sure and go to class, study and not to party too much. So weird, coming from Trenton. I have a home until Saturday and then I move to the Marriott. There was no guarantee that we would be able to stay there after the 30 days. That is about all for today. Thanks again for everything.

Email from Adam

Tell Trenton I will burn the DVD tonight and then get it in the mail to him tomorrow. It is a good movie and I will get it to him ASAP. If he has any request or any favorite movies I can go rent them and then burn them so he can have them for his enjoyment. It is no big deal so make sure he gives me some requests. The video store in town rents their DVDs for 87 cents so I can rent and burn as many as he wants. I miss you guys a lot and hope all is well

August 31, Tuesday, Update from Me

I know this is an early email but I did a lot of thinking last night. Again, this is my therapy so please let me vent. I will understand if you want to be off the email list when I am done.

I try to make the updates fairly light and will continue to do so but then I was thinking I am not doing Trenton any favors by sugar-coating this. Trenton was in a fairly bad mood last night and really had been except for the first hour when I got here last week. So I asked him why, when he has company, he seemed to be so much better. And, already knowing the answer, he told me that he could be himself with me. So, being the mature one, I stalked out of the room and took a walk within the hospital. I ran into Goldie and she was sitting in the hallway by the nurse's station and her timer was going off because she needed a weight shift so I asked her if she was ok and did her weight shift for her. She thanked me and yes, she is whiney, but poor thing, I would be too. They can't do anything for themselves. They can teach them to do their own weight shifts by puffing and sucking on a tube that is stuck in your face all day but you still have the timer going off and you have no way of turning it off or resetting it. You are literally reduced to being an infant again in an adult body. Trenton told me he wakes up at 4:00 in the morning feeling trapped in his body.

The #1 cause of paralysis is car accidents, then diving and ski accidents. But some are in here for something as innocent as falling off a chair while changing a light bulb.

Since the night was not quite stressful enough, Trenton gets a tech who has no idea what she is doing and he finally gets into bed around midnight. At that time we had a really good talk. He said that they have been telling him that if the nerves don't come back that it doesn't matter how much you work. I don't necessarily believe that, but I do know that the research and technology is out there to help regenerate those nerves, not only for spinal cord injuries but for Parkinson's, cancer, Alzheimer's and others. It is important to understand the type of research they are doing and do away with the misconceptions associated with it.

I'm sorry. I don't mean to preach but when you see someone you love or Goldie (who I don't know at all) struggle you want to do as much to help them as you can. Trenton is not feeling sorry for himself and he knows it could be worse, but he is struggling a bit. Thanks for hearing me out and I promise I won't do this daily.

On a lighter note, Trenton does not want to get up today so Angie, a very special nurse, came in with a KC Chiefs hat for him to try to cheer him up. They are awesome here for the most part and again, I can't thank all of you enough for the cards you send and your support.

Venting can be a good thing.

One of my faults is I can be somewhat immature. Such was the case the night that precipitated the above update. I had gotten my feelings hurt because you wouldn't talk to me. Now the rational person, and the one I aspire to be, knows the reason. I am your mother and you can be yourself with me. But, being rational was not happening. I got upset and said something to you and then you got upset. We got into an argument and I did what I do best, which was to walk away from the argument. This was the first fight we had since the accident. And I should have just let things go, but I had tried to talk to you and you weren't responding and I took it personally.

I realize I have joked in this book about my parenting skills. The truth is, even through those "horrible" years all teenagers go through, we basically got along. We had what I thought to be a pretty good relationship as you grew up. Most of that changed with this accident. I will start by saying I understand why it has changed. You don't want to be real open with me about your issues because you don't want me to worry. You also don't want me to try to "fix" anything. We have had several issues where I have listened to either well-meaning family members or your caregiver and I have panicked, which resulted in either me calling for an ambulance or building a wheelchair-accessible house. I know, a little extreme. The fact of the matter is, you want to make these decisions and you do not want your mother to get involved and you really don't want to live with your parents. But, let's just say that understanding why we don't talk does not make it any easier. Honestly, you don't share your feelings with anyone and, of course, I worry about that as well.

During your stay in Springfield you denied wanting or needing a minister or a therapist. You consistently said, "I don't need to talk to anyone." I attempted to see a therapist right after the accident and then about a year ago I saw one Angela recommended. That poor guy. I walked into his office and all he said was, "How can I help you?" and I started crying and didn't stop until the session was over. I went one more time and the same thing happened. I really liked him, but I was so exhausted after those two sessions from all the crying, I couldn't function for the rest of the day. He was supposed to get in touch with me for another session and I never heard from him. I am sure it was a misunderstanding as to who was to get in touch with whom, but I really don't think he knew what to do with me.

Well-meaning friends also thought it would be helpful for me, and especially for you, to meet others who had been injured. I met several wonderful people. The problem with this was the conversation revolved around your injuries and then I would be sad and depressed for the rest of the day. While you and I didn't discuss this, I am guessing you felt the same way. I needed as much normalcy in my life as possible. To this day, I talk about your injury very minimally to my friends. First of all, it does make me sad and I never know if I am going to be able to control myself. If someone does ask about you, I say you are good. If they ask me more questions and I can tell I am getting emotional I tell them either, "I don't want to talk about it anymore," or "I'm (he's) fine." They know me well enough to know I am not trying to be rude and no one gets offended.

I feel I am doing better. I know you must be thinking, "It's been ten years Mom." I know this. But, as you know, this is an injury that just keeps on giving. There is always something to worry about, and even if there isn't, I still worry. Initially, after the accident I kept incredibly busy. I have always been busy and very social, but this was ridiculous busy. I went back to school to get my Bachelor's. I wanted the Patient Advocate position at CMH and a friend of mine got the open position over me because she had a bachelor's degree and I didn't. So a year after your accident I did online classes and got my degree. I was very fortunate they hired me as a Patient Advocate. While I was getting my degree, I was still working as an Administrative Assistant and involved in Book Club, dinner groups (several) and well, you name it, I was doing it.

Had I lost my mind? In some ways I would say, "Yes." I couldn't be idle because I might think about you and it became difficult. I have moved three times since your accident. I would joke with my friends that I had a problem. The problem was everyone knew, including me, it was not a joke. I constantly needed something "new" to keep my mind occupied. I had to get a handle on it or I was going to go broke. I don't know if I have gotten better or not, but I am truly making an effort. I guess if nothing else, age will slow me down at some point. Also, having Madi, Emma and now Liam has helped me immensely. And, my job has helped. A lot of people thought I would be good at being a Patient Advocate. I had lived this and could relate, or so everyone, including me, thought. Unfortunately, I wasn't stellar at first. There were times I couldn't understand the complaints. It was hard for me at this point to understand how anyone could be upset over a two hour wait in the emergency room. But I got bet___ ___ly. I couldn't think about your situation and compare it. ___ ___yone has different coping skills and no matter wh___ ___ through, it is a big deal.

Email from Gerry

Susan,

My name is ___ry, I'm Kristi's aunt. I've met Trenton a few times. ___ met Trenton at a casino one night when he was with Kristi and so___ other of their friends. Tell him Kristi never got over being sooo embarrassed because I made him get up from the seat so I could play a penny machine.

He also came to my house for Kristi's graduation party.

He is such a sweet, kind and upbeat kid. My oldest daughter is mildly retarded and Trenton was so kind to her that day. She tends to talk a lot if she gets any attention.

He also played with my grandchildren, so I know there is something VERY SPECIAL IN HIM.

I went with Kristi to the prayer service for him and he is in my prayers every day.

Tell him Aunt Gerry said to please be strong as he has so much to give and so many people pulling for him. Anyone who is kind to special people, like my daughter Maria, and to children, is very special and is blessed with a special gift.

September 1, Wednesday, Update from Me

Hello.

Thankfully, no one asked to be off the email list. In fact, everyone was wonderful and I even wanted to call some of his friends tonight just to talk. Don't get me wrong; he is still bossy and demanding but I can deal with that. He has had some good news in that he is now on an unrestricted diet and, trust me, he is eating everything in sight, which means he is off the feeding tube as of tonight. With this new trach he has in he quacks or moos, not intentionally but the trach is very sensitive and if it gets dirty at all he literally quacks loudly. They hear him clear down the hall.

He had a great PT class today. Unfortunately, she was a sub, but both Trenton and I liked her a little better than his regular therapist. She just seemed to work him a little more. I was asking the Occupational Therapist how long after an injury you can expect sensation to come back and she said she had heard up to two years. I had actually heard longer but I think that was encouraging to both Trenton and me. Trenton's injury is a complete C4-5, which means he does not have any feeling below the injury, which in Trenton's case is about three fingers above the nipple. If it is an incomplete injury, for instance a C2 incomplete, it means you would have some sensation below the point of injury. There is a guy from Hawaii whose injury is that and he is going to be able to get off the vent, since it is an incomplete injury.

Some of you had mentioned that you had tried to go online to Adaptive Adventures to find Matt Feeney. Once you pull up the website it will say "Feeney Wins Prestigious Award" and click on it to read about him. He is supposed to come to talk to Trenton tomorrow.

Tomorrow is an outing and they are going to a museum and lunch. But tomorrow is also the sign up for the Broncos/Chiefs game here on September 27th. They only have three spots so I have to get down there early to sign him up.

Thanks again for letting me vent. Trenton wants to eat so I have to go.

Love, Susan

Email from Sam

Susan,

Thank you for being honest. You deserve to vent whatever way you see fit and Trenton has every right to feel down whenever he wants. What happened, it doesn't make any sense. I know that is why I get so angry when I think about his accident. It was unprovoked and is simply something no one should ever have to experience. I applaud you for your candor and your bravery helping Trenton. And I think the one amazing sign in this entire e-mail you wrote is that if Trenton isn't feeling sorry for himself and thinking it could be worse, then there is an incredible, undaunted, special spirit in his heart. That speaks volumes to me. Trenton's life is meaningful, Susan. I know you know that, but he may not. Your email spoke to me today, which is why I responded. Sorry if I said anything out of line. I appreciate your honesty. And as far as stem cell research goes, the people who are against it are against because no one they love has been hurt or has needed it. It would only take some hotshot Republican senator's son getting paralyzed and then he'd be all for it. If it is an option that you can explore, then please do. Also, is there anything you or Trenton need? I will be sending him some stuff probably towards the end of September to early November. Is there anything either of you specifically want? I'm gonna send some things for Trenton anyway, so if there is something, tell him to speak up.

P.S-Tell him those Chiefs looked good the other night.

Email from Jeff (a friend of ours)

Susan, I don't think Trenton would be human if he wasn't struggling or feeling a bit sorry for himself. I know if I was in his shoes, I would. I know it has to be extremely difficult for him, and you guys, to look forward to the future. And it has to be stressful to be there but even more stressful not to be. I know all the support you have been getting certainly helps but doesn't alter the situation or the long road ahead. I know our family is always thinking about you guys and wondering what more we can do to help. If you need to vent to all of us it is more than understandable. Let us know if you need anything at all.

If Jamie needs anything be sure and let us know. I hope school is going well for her. I am sure she is putting in long hours at the library :)

Email from Lindsay
Hey Susan-

Your recent email really touched me. I am not a mother, so I cannot even begin to understand what you are going through right now. Trenton is family to me, and I am hurting so much - I am sure your pain is unimaginable. When we were out there a couple weeks ago, I did feel Trenton was doing really well. But at the same time, there were times I would look at him and could tell he was asking so many questions in his mind. He just looked empty and sad - and I knew there was nothing I could do about that but be there. I imagine that he feels no one can understand what he is going through and it is hard for him to talk about. Please don't be discouraged by his attitude. As you know, and as many people have told you, he needs this time to grieve.

On the plane back to DC, I read *Nothing is Impossible* by Christopher Reeve. He was telling his story from the perspective of someone who was looking back at his survival of eight years. He talked about his depression, his family influence, his hopes, religion, etc... I really enjoyed this book, and think Trenton will later on. I encourage you to read it. I gave Trenton a copy when I was there, so it should be on his shelf next to the picture wall. It's a small book and won't take much time to read. I especially liked the chapters on Recovery, Faith, and Hope. And at the end there is a section called "Afterward" that was extremely insightful. Trenton is going to deal with this in his own way, so I in no way am comparing him to Christopher Reeve. It just helps to read such influential words in the light of someone who had it much worse than Trenton.

He may not say it, but Trenton likes having you there. You are someone he can show all his emotions to, even anger, which I am sure is coming out now. Take it one day at a time and know you have a trillion people there for you.

In your spare time, it would be helpful to call Bernadette. She is the senior information specialist at the Christopher Reeve Paralysis Resource Center. She can answer ANY question you may have regarding what Trenton is experiencing and how to get him home and on with his life. Please give her a call. I am going to email her now and let her know you may be calling. She is very, very sweet and knows EVERYTHING about paralysis. At the least, shoot her an email.

Email from Adam

Tell Trenton to eat more grilled chicken than pizza. It is better for him, lol. Man I miss him a lot. What do you mean by him quacking? That is awesome he is on a non-restrictive diet. Will he ever be able to move his arms again? Or does that seem unlikely? I have learned a lot about back injuries since Trenton had his. We had to learn about them for my job in case we deal with back injuries at work. I learned all about the C4 & C5; also about the lower lumbar area. As soon as our teacher started going over that stuff I had a million questions on it, so I can get a better understanding of his injury. She said, and I knew, it was a very serious injury. I really want to burn more DVDs for him, I will compile a list of what I have and send him the list. I miss you guys a lot. Keep strong and I am glad to hear you and he are doing much better.

These updates were my therapy. Whatever the day brought I knew I could write my update and I felt comfortable sharing for the most part. I certainly didn't want to share anything that would make you feel uncomfortable, but somehow it helped me knowing I had people willing to read my posts and take the time to write me back. I understood and understand everyone has their problems. Ours at that time just happened to be at the forefront. I didn't and still don't want to ever come across as whiny or feeling sorry for myself. Working at a pediatric hospital, you see and hear something terribly sad every day. I don't doubt we could all write books about our life experiences. But, with every update I wrote and with every response I received, it helped me get through the day and move on to the next.

Email from Meggie (a friend of yours)
Hey Susan,

First off, I don't think any of your emails are too long. I think that everyone loves hearing from you. Anyways, I was just wondering if the "smilebox" we sent Trenton was okay. I know it was full of candy and sweet stuff, but I thought it would be nice to have that stuff around just in case he wanted any. I'm sorry if it's not okay.

Email from Geralyn (a friend of mine)
Susan,

You and Trenton have every right to be going through what you feel. The anger is normal. Let's face it, this has totally fucked up all your lives and yes, things will never be the same again. As a mother, it would be insulting if Trenton didn't show his true feelings to you. He feels you are strong enough to take whatever he can dish out. That is a compliment. On the other hand, Trenton needs to get a grip on it and to let up a little when you are there. You are not his punching bag.

This may sound cold-hearted but you have to look at what went right. In short, I find it to be a miracle that Trenton was found before he drowned and came out of this with no brain damage. What are the odds of that! The research on spinal cord injuries is moving at a phenomenal pace right now and breakthroughs are happening every day.

I know you have heard a thousand stories and it seems we all have them. I lost my only brother in a car accident when he was seventeen years old. He died of a broken neck. Still, after 30 some years, I wake up from some awful nightmares. My parents never got over the loss and neither have my sisters and myself. The anger is always there and always will be; you learn to live with it. People would tell us his passing was for the best, think of what he would be like if he had survived and how hard it would have been on the family. I know to this day if my brother could have survived with his mind intact and we were capable of giving him a quality life and a will for life, there is nothing any of us would trade that for than not to have him at all.

So Susan you can bitch as much as you want to. That is what we are all here for and thank God you have something to bitch about!

Trenton, you will have a life. It will be what you want to make of it. Focus on the positive and remember we are all so grateful you are here. It is the mind that makes the man. Remember to be strong not only for yourself but for your family also. I don't think there is a one of them who wouldn't trade places with you if they could. The future still holds all the positive things for you, including a job, a wife, a family, a home of your own. It is going to be what you make of it. Keep the anger; it is good. Just give it a break once in a while and smell the roses.

Email from Nathan

Hi,

Well, we finally got the venue for the band finalized it seems. The Pub has been really shady with everything and so we needed to find a more secure place. So, now we are having it for free at the bell tower on campus. We are going to have a bunch of guys walking around collecting donations from everyone in the crowd. What we are hopefully finalizing this week is having a meet and greet "after party" at one of the bars. Hopefully, the Outback, but who knows?

I also wanted to get some information about some bracelets or something. People, random people too, have been coming up to me on campus asking if we are going to sell blue bracelets that say "believe" on them. I had no idea about these and I talked to Derick Hill and he said to ask you about them. So, how do I get some to sell to people on campus?

You know, to be really honest with you, I have found myself getting wrapped up in all this planning/work and I sometimes forget why I'm doing it all and how serious it all is until I read your emails and take a break to think about it all. Your emails help remind me and drive me to make this all work out. It reminds me what kind of help I need to do and not be discouraged. Trenton and I, we never really hung out a lot, but I just want him to know that I am doing everything I can down here for his foundation and I guess just do my part as a friend and fraternity brother. I want him to know that we all feel like we need to work hard for him because he is working hard for himself. Everyone is counting down the days until we all get to hang out again. Today, we got two huge dump trucks full of sand and put it in our basement for a party we are having. Some of the guys had an idea to make some things out of sand and take a picture of it to send to Trenton saying "Hey, Trenton would love this, he would think it was hilarious!" Obviously they wouldn't be the most appropriate things, but nonetheless, things just are not the same here without him.

Well, I guess that's about it. Just thought I would let you know what was going on down here and ask a couple of questions.

Email from Donna (Sam's mother)
Dear Susan,

Since Trenton's accident, I keep a holy candle lit for him. I wanted you to know the other night I lit one for you and Rick so that you're able to stay strong and keep going. I can only imagine what you're going through and wanted you to know I say a prayer for you all every morning and evening. Thank you for your nightly email. The folks I work with ask me first thing in the morning what you had to say. Trenton probably doesn't realize he has people rooting for him that he doesn't even know.

P.S. I can relate to how these kids can be sweet, nice and fun with their friends and then glare at you....

Email from Kay (friend of mine and your teacher)
I know that there are so many people here at school and who have graduated who are thinking and praying for Trenton every day. I know things might not look good now, but miracles happen every day, and it seems like from your emails that he is getting through

some of the procedures and such pretty quickly, which is a good sign. I do not know him very well, but I do know him...and every time my sister or I saw him, he always made us smile. He is a great person, and I am always praying for positive things for him. I just thought maybe since you have had a bad day you would like to hear that. Thanks for sending the emails. You seem like a very strong person, and I know Trenton is.

You deserve to vent and then some--feel free to go off any time to me, because you deserve it. You are an inspiration to us all. I have been so moved by the way you have stepped up and accepted such a devastating situation. I think of you and your family often and pray that Trenton finds a way to deal with everything, as does your family. It broke my heart to read that Trenton wakes up at four and feels trapped. It sounded just like my mother. She suffered a stroke two years ago and while she is only partially paralyzed, she is very depressed and not much fun to be around. She constantly wishes to be dead. Thank God for Prozac and my brother and sister, who live near her. I question myself every day after talking to my mother to see if I could have handled this or that differently to make a difference in how she feels. I can't imagine how hard it is to deal with face-to-face every day, especially when it is your son. I'm not sure it is possible to ever know what to do in a situation like this but I think you are remarkable.

Email from Ann (friend of mine)

Hi,

You are in my thoughts so often. I hope you are doing alright. I'm sure you are just drained sitting with Trenton every day. I remember when Robbie had his lung collapse in high school and then the follow-up surgery. I would try and chit-chat with him and run and get him food and be all encouraging. Except driving to the hospital and home I would cry during most of the drive. I know Trenton is working hard and doing his best but it's hell on the parent too. I know this should be about Trenton, but you are in my prayers too.

Wanted to drop a note about your outing to the lake also. It sounded like something Bob did with me when I was in the physical rehabilitation hospital almost four years ago now. I don't know if you remember, but I almost died from a serious case of pneumonia. After being flat on my back in a drug-induced coma for two months I had no muscles and could not walk or even lift my knees up from the bed. I was sent to the rehabilitation hospital and was there for two months before I could even walk a little.

Anyway, I became very comfortable in my routine and comfort of the hospital. I really didn't care about what was going on in the outside world. I was just trying to cope with my condition and therapy. The nurses were wonderful and spoiled me. The doctor finally told Bob to start taking me out on the weekend for lunch or whatever. I really wasn't interested. What if I have to use the bathroom or will everyone look at me in the wheelchair? I still was not walking and could barely transfer from the car to the wheelchair. The doctor pushed and finally we went out for lunch. That was when I realized I was withdrawing. I needed the push to be part of the world and want to work harder. Please understand my thoughts. I totally know Trenton has gigantic challenges ahead. But I was happy he went out and participated in the outing. It's important to be part of the world and not get too comfortable in your own thoughts all the time. I hope I explained that okay. Anyway...even if he doesn't want to see the guy with the dogs (which I didn't care about either) it will probably give him a moment where it isn't about him and his limitations.

I know what you were facing with the new tech. I always hated weekends because you would get these green aides and techs filling in. One time I had one that woke me up in the middle of the night for blood pressure and then couldn't figure out what it was. Or the ones that couldn't draw blood, ouch!

What is your situation with where you are staying? I have a niece that has a house in Denver. Would it help if I asked if she had an empty bedroom? She's a character and in her first year of medical school. She's only 32 and recently divorced.

P.S. You can vent ANY time you want!

Email from Beth (a friend of ours)
Susan,

We are all rooting for Trenton, and he is stronger than most of us. Do you know of any movies he may want or anything else? I don't know if you have a VCR or DVD player down there, and what movies he might not have that may make some time go by. Please let me know of anything I can send to make things better, even if just for a minute.

Email from Carolyn (a friend of ours)

Hi Susan,

I just read your latest email and had to fight the tears. I had been saving this email to respond to when I was able to think of some insightful words to share, but nothing would come to mind each day when I reread it. Nothing other than I'm so sorry that Trenton has been dealt this incredibly tough obstacle, but now it sounds trivial and hollow.

If only all of us who know Trenton and your family could wish the circumstances to be different, you would all be home getting stressed at each other for all the little unimportant things in life we tend to stress over. I can imagine how desperately you and Trenton would wish you could turn back the clock to when he and his friends were younger, or even just a few seconds before that fateful night when life was so much simpler and so full of the promise of a different kind of life for him. I would think that if Trenton did not struggle with these feelings, it would mean that he had had brain damage, wouldn't you? (My sense of humor). It's a blessing that he feels like he can be honest with you, Susan, because I would think it takes so much energy to keep these emotions hidden from others. And I imagine that talking about it is important to his healing process. He has probably learned to count on your reactions and sense of humor, which I find so amazing.

Please don't remove me from your email listing and never hesitate to email directly if you feel the need to vent honestly. Matt and I both tend to be good listeners, as well as understanding of others. That's one of the things I so love and appreciate about Matt, although it's a burden too, sometimes.

I am passionate about stem cell research and was before I personally knew someone who could benefit from it, like Trenton could. I cannot understand the individuals and groups who are so against it and yet call themselves compassionate and pro-lifers. How much more pro-life can you be than to try to help the people who are living and struggling with overwhelming conditions to give them hope of a better life? As you probably realize, Matt works for American Century, whose founder, James Stowers, also founded Stowers Institute. I don't understand why, but it appears we all must fight to see that this research is encouraged.

I've probably gone on enough for now, but I just wanted to send my thoughts back to you. Tell Trenton that we think about him every day and to keep fighting. You take care, too, Susan, and stay strong.

Email from Matt
Hi Susan -

I've been staying busy. Work usually takes care of that task on its own. I was attempting to start an online degree through Park University (haven't graduated yet), but it didn't work out this semester. Fortunately, they're eight week semesters rather than 16, so I'll be able to pick back up in a few months.

I work in the Business Retirement Services department. I work with 401(k)s, 403(b)s, Sep/Simple/Sarsep IRAs, boring stuff like that. I do all their investments and transactions. But I actually like it. It's more interesting than it sounds. And it's a very good company. Like Adam, I sit at a desk all day. I guess I've gotten used to it by now, but if it weren't for meetings and projects I'd probably go a lil' nutty staring at a monitor all day.

I can remember playing basketball with all those guys. It seems like forever ago. I love looking at those old pictures. If my mom can't find that picture of Trenton and I, I'll have her draw one up from memory. =) (Not really)

I have a friend that's interested in donating to Trenton's organization. Can you tell me how she would go about carrying this out? She went to high school with him. Her name is Amy.

Thanks Susan, it's good hearing from you too.

September 2, Thursday, Update from Me

Hi all,

Trenton and I went with Layton and Goldie today to the museum and IMAX theatre for The Living Sea. We had lunch first and Trenton chowed down on a cheeseburger and fries. I think I had told you that when I am in these classes with Trenton I look around and wonder what everyone's story is. So today I was sitting by Layton in the van and he told me he had been scuba diving and got the bends. He is from Hawaii and such a nice guy. He asked me about Trenton and how his spirits were and I asked how he was dealing with it because the night before I had just told Trenton that Layton seemed so upbeat so I was surprised when he said he didn't want to live at first. He has a C2 incomplete injury but he will hopefully be able to live vent-free. He then said he realized he needed to live for his two grown children and two grandchildren.

We got back and I had to rush down to the rec room where you can sign up for two outings for the month of September. Of course, Trenton wanted to go to the Chiefs/Broncos game, which is September 27th, and thankfully I was able to get him on the list. In the meantime, Matt Feeney had come to visit with him. He is a good looking, athletic guy who 17 years ago was at Craig from a diving accident and was 25 years old at the time. He is a para who started Adaptive Adventures for the disabled with a friend of his seven years ago. I think Trenton really enjoyed talking with him.

Tomorrow is our conference and his grandmother, aunt, uncle and cousins, plus some friends, are coming to visit him. He is looking forward to it and it should be a nice weekend here so they can get out some.

He thinks this update is too long and is wondering what I could be writing about, so maybe he is right and I am making them a little too long. He forced me to read this to him and he wanted me to tell you all hi and thanks also. He can't remember Springfield at all, so he keeps asking me who gave him what and he wants to thank everybody. We started making phone calls yesterday. He really appreciates everything you all have done so much, as we all do.

He says I need to feed him now and college football is ready to start. See what I mean about being bossy?

The "bends" as referenced in the above update, refers to a diver who surfaces too fast. The excess nitrogen will come out rapidly as gas bubbles. Depending on which organs are involved, these bubbles produce the symptoms of decompression sickness. The risk of decompression illness is directly related to the depth of the dive, the amount of time under pressure and the rate of ascent.

Email from Rick (father of one of your good friends)

Susan,

Give Trenton our best! Chris, Erin and Sam just left for Denver. They should be there late tonight.

For my part, let Trenton know that he's not going to squeeze by me this year in fantasy football. I plan on kicking his behind!!

Email from Chuck (a friend of yours)

Susan,

Do you know anything about these Sygen Treatments? "In a small pilot study, seven of the 16 people given Sygen improved from near total paralysis to being able to walk after one year." Sygen apparently works by improving the ability of nerves to remain alive after injury and makes surviving nerves better able to function, but has not yet (March, 1996) been approved. This is what Dennis Byrd took; he is the player that got paralyzed during a football game.

Email from Sean (a friend of yours)

Hey Susan, it's Sean. I was wondering if there was any way I could get a list of the movies Trenton has out there. I want to get him some but I'm afraid he may already have them. Please tell Trenton I said hi and to keep up the good work and he better wear his Chiefs jersey when he goes to the game! Thank you!
Sean

My response:

Hey Sean,

Here is the list of movies out here right now:

Spaceballs
The Best of Will Ferrell
Gold Member
Meet the Fockers
Caddy Shack
Van Wilder
Sin City
Old School
Run Ronnie Run
Dodgeball
Tommy Boy
Truman Show
Ace Ventura
Super Troopers
Robin Hood
Chappell's
Tombstone
Rush Hour 2
Catch me if you can
Oceans 11
The Rookie
24
Seinfeld Season 3
Rudy
Traffic
Seven
Swiss Family Robinson
Good fellows
Snatch
Three Kings
Kill Bill 1st one
Training Day
Dead President

Half Baked
Austin Powers
Men at Work
Christmas Vacation
The Great Outdoors
Napoleon Dynamite
Hitch
Man of the House
Girls Next Door
Something about Mary
Road Trip
Arlington Road
Can't Hardly Wait
Bourne Identity
The Rock
Pulp Fiction
Family Guy
Swingers
A Beautiful Mind
Italian Job
2nd season
Entourage
The Simpsons 1st - 5th
Ray
Hoosiers
Scarface
Be cool
Casino
Fast & Furious
Braveheart
American History
Reservoir Dogs
Black Hawk Down

He also mentioned last night that he wanted to get some books on tape. Just ideas. But he really doesn't want anyone to do anything. He said everyone has been so great and not to do anymore.

You are beginning to do a little better

September 3, Friday, Update from Me

Hello,

First of all I want to apologize to several of you. I'm sure you must have thought that I had lost my mind when you received the same update at least three or four times. Jamie finally called me and told me to quit sending her the update. I kept getting a non-deliverable message saying there was offensive material and they would not deliver it. For the life of me I couldn't figure out what was offensive about it.

Speaking of Jamie, she sent Trenton a care package of all MU stuff and included a Tiger Tail so we put it on the back of his wheelchair. It looks pretty cute.

We had a good conference today. Dr. Chi reported that Trenton was doing well in all areas. Getting off the vent, his anxiety level is almost nil and he is participating in outings, to name a few. Then his PT and OT reported that Trenton was doing better in class. He is watching, as are we, the education tapes related to spinal cord injuries. Donna, his OT, reported that Trenton promised to start driving his wheelchair, quit calling it stupid and if movement does come back they can always modify the wheelchair according to his ability. The respiratory therapist is here right now and changed his trach to the smallest size, which means if all goes well and no complications, he will have the trach out next week and the hole will close up within a day. All this means that Trenton will be ready to go home around the 26th or 27th of October. So you can imagine how much work we have to do to be ready for him to come home. But it is good work because we will all be so glad to have him back.

Trenton is in his chair with two blankets, the heat all the way up and the shades open so the sun is beating in on us. All of you know that I don't get hot very easily and I am roasting. Because of his injury his body does not regulate temperature so he is either hot or cold, not much in between, and more often than not he is cold.

Dr. Chi mentioned Trenton's three goals when he first arrived to Craig. They were to get off the vent, do as much as he can on his own and to walk again. I love this doctor in that he doesn't discourage Trenton at all, and in fact, seems rather optimistic. He also does not object to looking into other avenues for spinal cord treatment such as China.

I look at the wall with all the pictures of Trenton with family and friends and I am so thankful he is here. Thanks to all of you.

September 4, Email from Ashley (your sister)
Hello-

I spoke with Chuck today and he was happy to do these t-shirts for an extremely discounted price. Small world-- he owns the bar at Northwest Outback and is actually hosting the event that Nathan (from Trenton's fraternity) is organizing with the band and stuff. Pretty cool. Anyway the t-shirts are either white or blue, short or long sleeved or sweatshirts.
Prices:
white t-shirt- $4.00
blue t-shirt - $5.00
white long-sleeved t-shirt- $7.00
blue long-sleeved t-shirt- $8.00
blue sweatshirt- $13.50
white sweatshirt- $12.50

Basically what I told them to do was put the superman logo with the T in the middle on the back of both t-shirts and on the front of the shirt have the Trenton R. Baier Believe Trust Fund logo in the middle of the shirt. Michelle (Chuck's daughter) is the design person and is coming up with a couple ideas and then e-mailing to me and I will choose. So what I need is sizes what color, either long or short sleeved or a sweatshirt or both. Please do this ASAP so I can give them an order form and they can get these to us by the week of the event.

Email from Adam
I am so happy you are able to take Trenton to the Chiefs game. Of all things that he could do, I think that is the thing that he will

love the most. He is such a huge Chiefs fan. Man I really miss you guys. I am going to come down for his thing at O'Dowd's, so I will see you guys there before the wedding, which is that Saturday. The thing at O'Dowd's is on the 22nd of September, right? That is a Thursday? I am really happy too, that he met with Mike Feeney. Hopefully he has a good spirit about it and is able to get out there and do stuff. (I can't believe what is going on). I am going to cry so much when I finally see him and you. (Sorry I am venting now).

Susan your emails aren't too long and I love to read them. I want to know everything and want to do my best to stay involved. Ask Trenton what DVDs he wants, I can send whichever he wants, it is really no problem.

I am going home tomorrow and will try and call you guys this weekend. Whose cell # did you give me in the email? I have yours already and Trenton's. Is it the same one?

Stay strong out there and the best will come from it. Have fun at the Chiefs game, and GO CHIEFS! (It is sad because up here they are all Minnesota fans, and Minnesota sucks!) Love you guys.

My response to Adam
Hi Adam,

Sorry I am just now getting back with you. It has been crazy. When we found out he will be home by the end of October it put us into a bit of a panic mode. We need to figure out so many things, like where he is going to live and we have to order so much equipment. It is so overwhelming but it will be so good to have him home. I am home now because Jamie and Ashley's birthdays are this week and I wanted to celebrate with them. Chris is out there now and Ashley will be out there on Thursday. I will be back out on the 16th - 20th then back for the O'Dowd's. I am so glad you will be there for that. It will be great to see you. Please feel free to call us and you can talk to him or give me your # and I will call you when I get out there.

I know what you mean. I am an emotional mess all the time. But we do what we have to do. You will be fine. You have always been very special to me. You and Trenton were so cute when you were little. You with your blond hair and he was dark with those glasses. Everything will be ok, I just don't know when.

Hang in there and let me know if you want me to call or you call me. Love to you.

September 5 Update from me

Hi,

It is hard for me to write when I am not there and don't know firsthand what is going on. All I know is we are all in panic mode to get things ready for Trenton to come home. There is quite a bit to think about. If anyone owns a state-of-the-art (meaning voice activated everything), wheelchair-accessible home that they would like to sell, please call us immediately. Thanks to Cathy, we all went to Mark's house. He was injured in a diving accident a year ago and was at Craig. He is also a quad, and through the help of family and friends, they converted his house and added on a bedroom and bath for him. Through a headset he was able to open the door, turn on the TV, change channels etc. It really is amazing with the technology today what they can do. For his computer, he had a pair of glasses without the glass that has a dot in the middle of them and when using the computer he can stare at an icon and it will double click it. He is able to live relatively independently.

I talked to Trenton tonight and he is getting the trach out tomorrow, which is very exciting. He had a great weekend with his friends and family. He will get a different wheelchair tomorrow to see if he likes this one better and then if he does they will measure and order him one. Craig was also going to work with him on a voice activated phone and get his computer ready. Ashley and Tyson are going out Thursday to celebrate Ashley's birthday.

Email from Gloria

Susan, I met a man who knows someone who has had a spinal cord injury and did the stem cell. He is now using his hands after many years (not his fingers). I got his number and would like to call him for you and see if it is ok to give you the number for you to talk to him. Would you like for me to do this? I wanted to talk to you before I call him to make sure you wanted to talk to him. I think he can help you and Trenton. His accident happened when he was around Trenton's age and I think he is around 32 now. Please let me know if you want to talk to him. I always send my love and prayers.

Email from Nathan

Hi,

This is Nathan. I am talking to the band who is coming up to Maryville for the benefit concert for Trenton and the Reeve Foundation and I am working on getting him a CD and poster signed by the band. I don't have the address to send it to though. I can't find it. If you could email me that, it would be awesome. I don't know if you or Trenton have heard of them before but they rock. You can hear them on their website thesoundandthefury.com and click on psychofans part. I don't know if I gave that to you already or not but either way, there ya go again. Tell Trenton I said hey and that everyone down here is working hard to get the word out about his foundation.

Email from Sally (a friend of mine)

Hi Susan, Your emails are not too long! Without you, we wouldn't know how Trenton is doing! Please keep them coming. Regarding the wheelchair, I bet any wheelchair Trenton gets would be custom made for his specific needs anyway. My friend Pam's Uncle Bill was a quad. He has recently died. He was a quad from an accident. I believe he fell down some stairs. Her Aunt said if you want to talk (or vent) to someone who was somewhat in your situation, you may certainly talk to her. I think of you and Trenton every day and pray for you. Say hi to Trenton for me. Sounds like he's eating so much better now. Should we send some more peanut butter cookies?

Email from Dick (your uncle)

Susan,

I'm very impressed by your attitude and response to Trenton's condition. Your e-mails, which I have forwarded from Annie, all seem positive, yet realistic.

Please hang in there as you have this last few months. You have been an inspiration for the rest of us, all of whom will face some obstacles in the future, and we can learn from you.

Email from Sammy

Susan:

I talked to my friend who works for Remax and he's come across some homes that are accessible; he's going to send me an email of listings and I'll forward them to you.

It was really good to see Trenton finally. I hadn't got to see him since Springfield, and this is the first time I've had a conversation since the accident. He was in really good spirits and joked around the entire weekend. He let me help with lunch and dinner several times this weekend, which surprised me because I didn't know if he would be comfortable with that. To be honest, I was hesitant at first. I helped him finish a Little Debbie snack. On Saturday, Chris, Erin, and I got him a spicy chicken sandwich from Wendy's. He said it made him feel extremely warm, which was a good thing (who would have guessed Wendy's restaurant could help increase internal temperature). He also let me help with weight shifts since his wheel chair was messing up.

You could tell that he was glad to see all his friends that visited, especially Chris. They did fantasy draft over the phone with Chuck, and Trenton is certain that he has a good team for the fantasy league. Some of his friends from school brought him a Royals-Build-A-Bear, which he liked a lot also.

Anyways, it was great seeing him. I was shocked at the progress he's made so far, and according to the nurses, he has a very busy week ahead of him. As always, if I can do anything, please let me know.

Email from Janine

Hi Susan

I was watching **Entertainment Tonight**, either Thursday or Friday, and they were interviewing this Asian guy who used to be on the show **21 Jump Street** with Johnny Depp. This guy's wife was in a car accident and is paralyzed (not sure the extent of it), but anyway, she is one of only three people in the US who has had stem cell treatment and now has movement she didn't have before. You may want to check out ET's website and see if they have any info on her. Not sure if you can contact her or contact her through ET but it might be interesting to see how she got on the list for the cells and how much mobility changes occurred due to the stem cell.

September 6 Update from Me

Hi all,

I just got off the phone with Trenton and he sounded great. He did not get the trach out as planned. He said everyone was telling him he was getting it out today except Dr. Chi, who has to write the order for it. Apparently, Dr. Chi wrote the order today so he will get the trach removed tomorrow. He should also get the neck brace off within the next several days, which makes a huge difference in how he looks. They put him in a different wheelchair today. He said the one they put him in today was easier to drive and he just liked it a little better. I imagine they will now measure him and get him one ordered. Unfortunately, he has had a lot of nerve pain, mostly because he hadn't been to PT for five days with the outing Thursday, conference Friday and then the holiday weekend. Hopefully, some stretching will help with that. He had just gotten his dinner so we did not talk long but he did say that I needed to look into voice activated phones because he had a lot of phone calling to do to thank a whole lot of people. I told him I would get right on it.

I will let you know if the trach comes out tomorrow. Thanks for everything.

Email from Kurt (neighbor and friend)
Susan: Babs asked me if I knew of anyone who might do some conversions at home to make things a little easier for Trenton. I contacted Ron, who owns a company called Automated Lifestyles in Gladstone. He mentioned Honeywell was developing some advanced technology–voice recognition. Ron has products that can do things by touch. I don't know if either of those might be appropriate with Trenton's condition. Anyway Ron will look into what might be "out there".

September 7 Update from Me

Hi all,

My phone rang tonight and it was Trenton. I had called him about 4:00 their time and Diana, who works at the front desk, said that he had just left for therapy, which was later than normal. I asked if he was driving by himself and she said he sure was. He had been all over the place. So he used Courtney's cell phone and called to ask me where Ashley and Tyson were. He was thinking today was the 8th. Anyway, he did get his trach out. He said it went well, really not a big deal and that it was easier to eat, talk etc. His chair is easy to drive and took him a day, just like he said it would take him. I think he was disappointed that Ashley and Tyson weren't going to be there tonight, so of course then I ramble on about the time they will be there tomorrow and Rick will be there on his way back from Vegas and I will be there the 16th and then every week until he comes home. Kind of like I'm doing now. Then Jamie calls and tells me it is parent's weekend next weekend when I am in Colorado and I feel bad about that. I think I need some major drugs! Honestly, I am joking.

I do appreciate all of you with information for us regarding equipment for Trenton and also information on stem cell studies. With Ashley and Tyson there tomorrow I should have more to share with you.

Email from Nathan

Also, I am new to this whole benefit concert stuff, but usually they have someone talk before the show who is close to the foundation. Since you are coming up, I am sure that people would love to hear what you have to say about how everything is going. You could introduce the band too. So, let me know what you think. Obviously, you don't have to, but it's an option that is there for you if you or anyone else would like. Just let me know.

Email from Sandra (friend of ours)

Hi, Susan:

I just returned from vacation to this good news about Trenton's progress. Congratulations to all of you! This is wonderful news.

This is also remarkable that he will be able to be back here in October. Does this mean he will be at your home or will he go to a rehab facility first?

Based on what Jeff has told me, this is truly amazing that he is doing so well this soon. I think Jeff was at Craig for nearly a year! And his injury was a T/ 7 - 8 or so. Good work!

Thanks for including me in your updates. I will continue to send best thoughts for all of you and to hold you in my prayers. I'm sure you cannot imagine how your life has changed and of course, for Trenton, most of all.

I'm so glad I got to spend time with you, your daughters and Lindsay. What terrific young women they are and how wonderfully they have risen to this most difficult occasion. Someone once said, "What doesn't kill us makes us stronger." Wow, how much can we take at times?

Email from Libby (friend and member of LNO)

You would never be able to remember your schedule with major drugs! Susan - Hey - how was Ladies Night Out (LNO)? Annie and I had to miss because of open house at school. Did you all plan a date for October? Love your updates - but I get confused when you are talking about "Rick" which one is it - Rick I or Rick II?! Sounds like Trenton is doing terrific. Don't worry about parents weekend - it is our Dad's weekend and Allen can't go either......there will be other years. Besides - it is Parent's Weekend for the entire university - ADPi may be having another Parents Weekend on their own - or a mom's or a dad's weekend separately - you can ask Jamie that.

My response to Libby

No, I am fine on drugs. Just sort of joking, but they are nice when you need them. We missed you last night. Our next one is October 20 at Ted's Mountain Grill in Zona Rosa. How is everything else going?

Email from Judy Vuagniaux (friend and member of LNO)

Is that my cue? (Drug rep) I still have 7 Xanax left and I only need 1-so you are welcome to the other 6. When is the next LNO and where? I will be seeing Jane tonight at tennis- I can leave her with the Xanax.

In the beginning of this book I said I had a strange sense of humor. These updates went to a lot of people, some I had never met and others I knew, but not well. I would forget they might be reading some of my comments and take me literally. I was not sedating myself. I took the one antidepressant daily that I started when I got to Craig and that was it. But, it was nice to know I had people who could hook a brother up!

Approximately 35 years ago another friend of mine from the neighborhood created a group and we named it Ladies Night Out. It has evolved in the 35 years, but the core group has stayed together. As you can imagine we have been through a lot in the 35 years we have been together.

Email from Clifford

Miss Baier,

My name in Cliff. I am one of Trenton's friends from school. I currently am a Project Manager. If there is anything you need to have done to make your home accessible for Trenton I would be glad to help as far as ramps, widening doorways or accessibilities issues in the bathroom. I work a lot with ADA standards so I know what will probably need to be done. Regardless of whether you decide to move or not I would love to help out because he was a very dear friend to me. Let me know what I can do and I'll see about getting it done.

My response to Clifford

Thanks so much for the offer. Right now we are looking at a house across from Eastgate Middle School that the North Kansas City School District built for the disabled. I think it would be perfect but haven't seen it yet; hopefully this weekend. I will certainly keep you in mind. We thought he would be coming home the end of November and we are thrilled that he will be coming home earlier, but there is just a lot to get done.

Thanks again and I will keep you posted. I will also let Trenton know you wrote. He is so appreciative, as we all are, of everyone's generosity.

Making plans to come home

Y ou wanted to live on your own with a couple of your buddies. It wasn't that I was against this idea; it was that I didn't see how it was going to work. Rick was working on finding you a place to live. You needed a roll-in shower and wider doors for easy access at a minimum. We had a small selection to pick from and not much time. We also needed a wheelchair accessible van, shower chair, Hoyer lift and as much voice activation as we could afford. As you can imagine, none of this was cheap. We ultimately found a maintenance free home in a retirement area. The bathroom needed to be reconfigured a little bit to accommodate you, but otherwise was perfect. You have been there ever since and it really has been a perfect house for you.

Email from Rebecca (daughter of a friend of mine)
Hi Susan!
This is Rebecca, Faith's daughter. She has been keeping me updated on Trenton. Please know that he is in our thoughts and prayers. I am so sorry that I have not emailed you sooner. Starting this school year was kind of hectic. I have Pre-K students with developmental delays, and we are so much lower than we were last year! It has definitely taken some adjusting to meet their levels. Anyways, I am so glad to hear that Trenton is on the pathway to get home. I am also so proud of his accomplishments. I have shared his story with a few friends down here, and they are also amazed at how far he is coming along. Please let him know that I am thinking of him. We are in the works to send him something from our class. I guess it really needs to get mailed, as it looks as though he could be going back home soon! If there is anything that I can do from Jacksonville, Florida, or if you know of any places where I could get you information, even though it seems like you are on top of things, please don't hesitate to ask. Thanks for keeping us updated on

Trenton and tell him that there is love coming from Florida!

My response to Rebecca
Hi Rebecca,

It is so nice to hear from you. How are you doing and how do you like Jacksonville? I am sure you are enjoying your work but it sounds fairly challenging. I am so proud of how all you kids turned out. Notice how I still call you "kids." I see Ryan every now and then at Tommy's and he is so sweet and personable.

I am also proud of Trenton. He obviously has some bad days but for the most part he really has stayed focused and determined, which is why I think he has progressed so much and so quickly. Trust me, we were a little shocked to find out he will be coming home late October. We were thinking late November. We are thrilled, but there is a lot to do. It certainly has been hard on all of us but I know we will be ok eventually. I tell everyone we are just redefining "normal" and honestly, our family wasn't all that normal to begin with.

Thanks again for writing, so nice to hear from you. Take care of yourself and please keep in touch.

Email from Linda and family (friend of ours)
Dear Susan,

I know that you have been busy with all of the therapy, treatments, plans of care, etc. Just know that Trenton, you and your family have been in our thoughts and prayers. We have also prayed for Trenton each week where I am currently working.

It seems that Trenton is making progress each day. I'm sure there are good days and even a few that are not so good. I guess that is a part of the journey.

I want you to know that if there is anything I can do or Mike can do, we will be there for Trenton and for you.

I'm sure there will eventually be a transition back to Kansas City. Please call if you need anything.

We like the emails from Annie that keep us informed. Hopefully doors will continue to open.

Email from Chris (friend of mine)

Susan,

I don't really know how to say this or word it without sounding like I'm butting in, so I'm just going to say it straight out.

I work with a lady whose mother is wheelchair-bound. I was asking her how she went about preparing the house her mother lives in. Apparently she had it built when the situation arose, but she has learned a lot of stuff over the years and has had to figure it out on her own. She lives up north and says she would be happy to come over and give you ideas or suggestions on what modifications you could have done to your house or just talk through anything that would help you prepare for Trenton's arrival home. She's not pushy or know-it-all in any sense.

If you have any interest, let me know and I'll put you in touch with her. If not, that's fine too.

It sounds like things are progressing well for Trenton and I can't wait to hear that the trach is out and the brace off. He's a very lucky young man to have such a great mother.

Email from Mary Alice Morrissey (friend of mine)

Dear Susan,

You write such wonderful e-mails and we very much appreciate the updates. Each day is a new experience, I'm sure, and for those of us who can't be there it helps to be updated. Please don't feel you're boring anyone. If anything, more information would be better.

I only knew Trenton as a young boy. I know Jenny liked him and I value her judgment. I see his personality through your updates. I love his determination and spirit. It will take him far.

When the girls had their (4) ACL surgeries, Jenny had her thyroid removed (in high school), Ed had his brain tumor surgery and prostate cancer, it hurt so much to see them pushing through the pain and working so hard to get better. Trenton will never believe this, but sometimes it's harder on the one watching. I don't mean to be trite and compare their injuries to his, but as a mother, I hurt to see the girls hurting and I had no means to help them outside of praying and doing little things to help. They both were nasty to me at times; I think angry that none of us could get how much they hurt but I know that they didn't mean to be mean. They just had to vent. I'm sure Trenton has that also, but I always knew that they loved me and knew that I loved them, and that's what counts.

I think of all of you daily. I pray for you daily. We will SOOOO celebrate when you all head home.

Email from Allison

Hi Susan, Sorry I have been unable to write for a week or so. Sounds like everything is still progressing for Trenton. Getting the neck brace off and trach out are huge things. I'm sure he is really looking forward to that. Will the bones in his neck be healed then?

I am assuming that you are in KC? Are you working and catching up on things? I meant to write you and tell you not to take me off the email list, but I figured that if you didn't hear from me that meant that you wouldn't. I don't mind hearing the good, the bad, and the ugly. I know this is hard for you and Trenton and the rest of the family. It's a grieving process---and you all have to go through all the steps. I definitely want to continue supporting you and Trenton and the rest of the family in any way I can.

So Trenton will be going home sooner than planned? Is that good? Will he be heading to one of your houses for a while before he plans on getting a place of his own? Knowing Trenton, he will be ready for his independence as soon as he can get it. I can't wait to see him and talk to him. I figured that he wouldn't remember Springfield at all. I will never forget seeing him and the smile in his eyes and him grinning so big to show me the missing tooth!! He isn't going to be able to make his fundraiser, is he?

You can pass this email along to Trenton, as always. I didn't know if he'd been following the Hurricane Katrina news or not. I'm sure you've told him about the kids we got from New Orleans. That was a crazy night! I'm so glad that he was in a hospital where he was and not anywhere close to there, can you imagine that! Anyways, Children's Mercy is taking volunteers to go to field hospitals anywhere from the Astrodome to Mississippi to New Orleans. I signed up, and will be working somewhere for two weeks in primitive conditions. We will be sleeping in tents and sleeping bags. I don't have a lot of information though. They just said they will call you 2-3 days before you leave and the government will get you where you need to be. I could be going the end of this week to next month. The relief process for these people is going to be a long time. Well, I just thought that would be some interesting news to tell Trenton.

Tell him I still think about him daily, especially every time I leave my parents' house. I wish I could've made it out there to see him, but it sounds like he'll be home sooner than later. Tell him the progress sounds good and he sounds like he's working hard. Many prayers are still coming his way.

Email from Adam
Hey Susan have Trenton call me whenever he has an opportunity. I am kind of nervous to call him, so have him call me please.

Love you guys. I have to get to work

September 8 Update from Me
Hello,

Ashley and Tyson got there about 2:00 today so they went to Trenton's last Tetra class. This was about 4 weeks of classes that dealt with lots of issues, from how to fly on a commercial airline with your injury to respiratory care. For today's class they (Goldie, Layton, Jerry and Trenton) were to come with a question. The panel members were three individuals with varying degrees of injuries who had been patients at Craig several years ago. I don't know what Jerry's question was and Layton's was somewhat personal so I won't get into that, but Goldie's question was "How do I accept what has happened to me?" By the way, her accident was caused by a drunk driver, which would be very hard to accept. Goldie is probably in her mid-60s. Ashley said by the time anyone could hear what her question was and then they started talking about it, Goldie had fallen asleep. Trenton wanted to know what to expect when he got home. I don't know what their answer was but Trenton said he wanted to do a lot more than they had said he could do, which sounded good to me. Ashley says Trenton is driving great, maneuvering through doorways, elevators etc. I asked him how it felt without the trach and he said it was much easier to eat, drink, talk etc. So in honor of Ashley's birthday and getting the trach out they were ordering Italian food and watching football tonight.

I know I am pushing it here a bit but remember when I asked if any of you knew of anyone who had a house totally wheelchair accessible etc.? Well, someone actually did. Well, now we are looking for a van with a chair lift. And, one other little thing. If anyone knows of a great, dependable, 24-hour caregiver that would love to be at Trenton's beck and call, well then, I think we would just be about set.

Email from Jo Ann (friend of ours)

Susan,

I don't know if anyone has told you about Doug. He is Julie's husband. She is a teacher at Antioch Middle School. He is a quad and has been since he was about 16 (I think). If you would like me to, I will contact them. They live in Liberty and they may have some good ideas for housing and caregivers. Trenton and your family are always in our thoughts and prayers.

September 10 Update from Me

Hello,

Ashley said Trenton was doing well. In OT they went across the street to a little sandwich/ice cream place yesterday. They took a little jaunt around the hospital and ran into Cindy, who went to Winnetonka and now works at Craig. She was talking to Trenton and suggested that he try to get to know some of the other patients who, like him, were going through some of the same things he was. This was good coming from her so Trenton had Ashley go down and look at the activities board to see if there was another outing he might like to go on. Next Friday when a bunch of us are out there, there is a BBQ and live band so he wants to do that. Ashley says he is in pretty good spirits and he certainly sounds good on the phone.

Somebody is pretty sneaky. Trenton has received an autographed Cardinals cheerleader picture and yesterday he received a New England Patriots paper with the cheerleaders cheering him on.

There is no return address and nothing to give us a hint as to who is sending all this. Trenton wants to thank you. All the males out there, including doctors, techs and nurses, have been admiring all his autographed cheerleader pictures.

I asked him if he was going to wear his Chiefs stuff tomorrow and he said "definitely."

I also want to thank you for your responses to my request for a van and 24 hour help for Trenton. This is such a great help to us. We can't thank you enough.

Email from Ryan

Hello Susan,

I feel like I should re-introduce myself since we have only really met via email. My name is Ryan and Trenton and I are good college friends. I am always very eager to get online to read about Trenton's progress (I really appreciate your honesty when you write your emails). I am a second year Physical Therapy student at KU Med (which is a third year grad program). But anyways, I am writing to see if you are still looking for any type of equipment to make your home accessible for Trenton. I thought that I could ask some of my PT professors at KU Med to see if they have any contacts. It is worth a shot to ask. I have talked to some of my professors about Trenton and they all say that Craig Hospital is the best. So I know that Trenton is getting the best care in the world. Let me know if I can help out in any way. Talk to you soon.

September 11 Update from Me

Hi all,

I just picked up Ashley and Tyson at the airport. They had a great time with Trenton. So much so that she said they almost missed their flight today because it was so hard to leave him. She said he was busy with his fantasy football and she suggested that tomorrow night he go watch Monday night football with some of the other patients. It was somewhat hard today to be at the game, just because I knew Trenton would have loved to have been there. I know he will get to a game sometime when he gets back.

I haven't had a lot of time this weekend but I very much

appreciate all the feedback on vans, 24 hour care etc. I am not ignoring you and I promise I will write you back tomorrow.

As some of you may have heard, Trenton wants to live on his own with a couple of roommates so we are looking at the house across from Eastgate Middle School that the North Kansas City School District built that is a wheelchair assessible house. It would be perfect but the only drawback is the sewers aren't in and they have been working on it with the city for about two months now and worst case scenario, it could be another six months, so we are hoping this gets worked out.

The O'Dowd's event is definitely September 22nd and more information should be coming your way soon. As always, thanks so much for your emails. It is always so nice to hear from you all.

Email from Krista (friend of yours)

Hey Susan

As you know we are coming up this weekend. I wanted to bring Trenton some things. What size T-shirts is he wearing these days, a large? Also, does he like any kind of cookies or treats? I thought since he was eating better he would enjoy some homemade cookies! Anything else you can think of that he might like or need? Also, if there is anything you need I would be happy to bring it with us. Is it too late to give pictures to Tyson? I found a few I would like to include in the show. Thanks so much and we can't wait to come visit!

Email from Janis (Aunt of Springfield patient we met while you were there)

Hi Susan,

It appears David is going to Rusk in Columbia, MO next Wednesday. Carolyn toured the facility today and is very pleased with it. Someone she talked with previously worked at Craig Hospital. They are looking at a 40 day stay but if he needs to stay longer the doctor will get the approval from the insurance company. They also told her that 90% of their clients go home and of the ones more like David, 75% go home, which is good news to us. Which will be interesting when the time comes there -- just family issues.

The nurses at Overland Regional are ready to kick the stepmom out -- I gather she is rude, confrontational, and difficult to communicate with and they are just tired of dealing with her and his dad ...what a mess.

How is Trenton this week? Have any of his friends been able to come and see him while he is out there?

How are you? Are you holding up emotionally? Mentally and physically?

Email from Denise (friend of mine)

Brian is doing better than me. He had blood tests yesterday for blood counts. He has one more session of chemo and then back to Houston on October 15. We are going to Mizzou's first home game this weekend so it will be interesting to see how he interacts with his frat brothers or even if he will go over to the house. I think he will.

UMKC is going OK. How hard for a kid to be independent doing what they want, when they want, and poof, it's gone. I'm sure Trenton and Brian could talk hours about this subject.

As for me, I'm half OK. I need to go to Houston and hear that the chemo and radiation are working. Chris is back in the swing of work and doing his work thing. As you know, it's just hard.

When are you going back to Denver? Again, one day at a time.

Email from Lisa

Hi Susan.

I'm not sure how serious you were being when you were asking about a caregiver but I just thought that I'd let you know that I would be more than willing to help out. I went to high school with Trenton and am dating his friend (Chase). Currently I work at NKC Hospital as a nurse tech while I get through Paramedic school (which will be in May). Obviously I am NOT available 24 hours a day but I thought I'd offer my help whenever it may be needed. I am certified in a lot of areas--CPR, ACLS (advance care life support), etc.--and have worked at the hospital for three years now. Just let me know...and if not, no biggie. Just thought I'd offer.

PS. I'm good friends with Allison ...we could gang up on Trenton and both of us help him...ha ha.

Email from Wayne & Shirley (your aunt and uncle on your grandmother's side)

Susan,

Be sure to tell Trenton that we are very proud of him for learning to use his w/c so quickly and for getting the trach out. I'm sure it is more comfortable for him. That will be great to have Ashley and Tyson out there. Don't feel guilty about not being at Jamie's for parents' weekend. She should understand and so should her friends. I hope she is getting along okay in college. I'm sure you get really spaced out with all that is coming towards all of you each day. They don't write books about things like what you are going through. Just remember we are all praying for all of you. Hope you can find a place for Trenton to live in KC that will be comfortable for him. Keep up the good work. I am still a Bronco fan, Trenton. Sorry. That goes back to when my nephew Dan got killed in CO and he was such a Broncos fan, so from then on, they have been my team.

Take care. Susan. You need to put all of these email journal entries in a book so you can go back and read them someday. Hope you have been keeping them.

Email from Nikki (your high school friend)

Susan,

Hello! I hope you are doing okay! I got the best surprise ever when I got home last night. I was checking my messages and was almost floored when I heard Trenton's voice on the machine! I was so excited I felt like a little kid who just found out they were going to Disney World. I called him back and we talked for about 15-20 minutes and he sounded so completely normal it was GREAT! He told me all about Craig and what he was doing and how he was ready to start his therapy in the pool soon, etc. He was also so sweet and thanking me for everything, I know he probably gives you a hard time a lot (I mean, come on, it is Trenton) but like they always say, you are toughest on the ones you love the most and with him that is definitely YOU! Although Trenton is a "quad" as he put it, it is sooooo wonderful to still hear that good old Trenton on the other end of the line and to know that this experience has not really truly changed the person he is.

You are doing an amazing job with everything that has been thrown at you in the last couple of months and I hope you know how good a person you truly are. You are so selfless and giving and I can only hope I will one day be as good of a mother as you are!!!! Thank you so much for always keeping us updated with news about Trenton! Take care!

Email from Chyleen (friends of the Baier's)

Susan,

I sent two packages to you today, UPS. They should arrive Monday. The baby quilt should bring at least $50 and the wall hanging $15-20. It just depends on who is there. But whatever they bring is fine with me. They are from all of my family: Evelyn, Lavon and Lyle, Shirley and Evan, Chyleen and Paul, and Gerald and Margaret. Please let Rick know that we sent them.

I want to tell you that we have such a great admiration for you and what you have done to help Trenton. You must be one of the greatest mothers ever. Your e-mails are so appreciated by us. You sound so positive and optimistic, which must be difficult at times. Anytime you want to vent and go the other way, please do so. We will all listen, say an extra prayer for you, and try to do something to help.

My son Andrew will be 24 on Monday and I don't think I could handle what you have. But moms dig into that supply of love and strength when needed, and somehow God helps them, and they know just what to do or say.

A week or two ago, when I was in Fontanelle, I met up with Jamey, a young man from Bridgewater, and I can't remember his last name right now. He is paralyzed from a high school wrestling accident about ten or more years ago. He owns a house in Fontanelle and is active on a number of projects. He is such a nice young man, has a positive attitude, and helps a lot of people. I see him occasionally at the nursing home, bringing joy and conversation to the elderly people there. I am always inspired when I see him, and he is always so pleasant.

I could easily do a couple of days a week as caregiver. I did a lot of this work for the Visiting Nurses in Iowa City and at a retirement home there. But we are probably a little too far apart, and with gas prices the way they are, for me to come that far. But keep me in mind for a substitute. I train easily to the patient's ways of wanting things done. I just never got a certificate in Kansas after I moved here. We live on the west side of Wyandotte County, near the Speedway.

I really do look forward to meeting you someday soon. I am sorry we will miss the benefit. I hope it is a successful event.

If there is anything that we can help you with, please ask. You are in our prayers, and my God bless you in all that you do.

September 12, Monday, Email from Sammy
Hi Susan,

It sounds like you are doing well and Trenton too! I was hoping that you could say hi to Trenton for me and tell him that I am very proud of him. My family and I continue to pray for you and your family and that I love him and miss hanging out with him.

And enough with the wishy washy stuff......How about that Chiefs game?! We looked pretty damn good, didn't we? I think that we made a statement yesterday and that we're a lock to win the AFC West and possibly the AFC! I had my shirt off at the game like a white hog....I'm pretty sure my family would have liked to disown me after that one. I can't wait to see you at O'Dowd's. I seriously am so proud that you are doing better. Congratulations on getting the trach out and coming so far. It will be nice to hear your goofy-ass laugh again. I know that you will continue to make everyone proud by working so hard and being positive. Have a good day Trent!

Email from Gloria and family
Susan, I looked into nursing care for Trenton and a friend of mine owns a place called Able Care. They furnish hospital equipment and another friend of mine said she thinks he can furnish nurse care. Susan, if you call, it is out north and tell him I sent you to find out if they have nurse care and I think he will help you with the cost.

The young man I told you about that was in the accident is Barry.

He is the young man that had the stem cell. Susan if you talk to him tell him that I was the one who left the message on his mobile phone. Good luck. I hope some of this can help you. If you need anything just let me know. Tell Trenton we all send our love.

Email from Glenda (friend of mine)

Hey Susan,

Guess you enjoyed the Chief's game, especially since they won. Tom and I listened to most of it on the radio while we were shuffling some of his trailers around for this week's sprinkler jobs. We had hoped to get up to the lake over the weekend but never made it there. You probably heard that I "crashed" the boys lunch date at Stroud's on Friday. I tried to get out of it but Tom insisted that I tag along. I am still not sure exactly why, but the food was great (as usual) and it is always a good time to be around those guys!

Tom and I would like to send Trenton something but what do you suggest? Is there a DVD he would like to have or what other ideas? Let me know.

It is good to hear that things are really progressing with Trenton and his attitude seems really good. Your family and all your friends are really being supportive, which I know is your saving grace. I swear I have never seen Ric 2 so mature - he has really stepped up to the plate here and I know you count on him for lots of things. It is good that he has some connections too.

Take care and we will try to get together with you guys when you have some time. I know you have lots of people pulling on your coat strings right now. Hang in there. We love you guys!

Update from Me

I just got off the phone with Trenton. John, his friend who lives in Colorado, is there watching Monday night football with him. He sounded good. His only complaint was a lot of nerve pain, which is normal but can be quite painful. He said his classes went well today and he is excited about his company this weekend. This is not going to be one of my more interesting emails, as when I am not with him there just isn't as much to write. So my emails this weekend should be great!

Hope everyone got the information on the O'Dowd's event. If you did not, please let me know and I will forward it to you.

We all are busy arranging for his homecoming and again thanks so much for all your feedback. It has been so helpful.

Email from Jane (my sister)

Susan, I know Rick is impossible to talk to but I had another thought. North Kansas City is building another house this year. If the sewer problem is not going to be resolved for a while, you might want to consider contracting this new house. It should be ready in May. Trenton could then get exactly what he wanted in it. Of course I guess you could do that on your own by just building any house. Just a thought. If you need me to talk to Dick to see about what the problem is with the sewers, let me know. Jim also knows Anita well. You know what kind of influence she has around here.

Email to Jane

We thought about that house but I guess we are going to see what they can do with this one. They don't want anyone to talk to the city as they have a good relationship with them and don't want anyone else involved. They seem to think it could be resolved soon. Rick did say he would start working on this so it is a waiting game.

Email from Amy (a friend of mine)

Hi,

I didn't get anything about the O'Dowd's event and I don't mean to pester you, but I'd like to send out a big email to all of my KC friends and encourage them to go. I wish we could go, but we're not going to be in town that weekend. Plus, I'm pregnant with Number Two (!) so I wouldn't be able to drink and whoop it up anyhow. :) I'm due beginning of April, so our kiddos will be about two years and two months apart. We'll be busy!

P.S. Just send me a quick email when you have time about the time, date, location, purpose, anything you have about the O'Dowd's event and I'll pass it along.

Email from Kristen (a friend of yours).

Susan, I have been getting the updates on Trenton and I saw that you needed some information on vans and lifts. I talked to a medical transporter and he said that the cheapest route would be to buy a van and then have a lift installed. The company that he uses is Handicap Conversions. He thought that you could buy the lift and have it installed for $5,500.00. He said that he has done a lot of research and they are the cheapest around and they do good work. Hope everyone is doing well, Trenton and your family are in my thoughts and prayers daily.

The list is long and continues to grow on what you need.

September 13 Update from Me

Hello,

I just got off the phone with Trenton and he is in bed, as he has an ever so slight beginning of a bed sore. He said they suggested he stay off of it tonight because he wanted to be good for this weekend. I'm a mess when no one is there with him, but he seemed good. I only rambled a little about when I was going to get there, exact time, etc. Of course, he is well aware of who all is coming out this weekend but I reminded him and I will repeat all of this the next two nights until I get out there. Thankfully, he knows how I am and just lets me talk.

Again, if you didn't get the information for the O'Dowd's event, I will be happy to send it to you.

We all have assignments since there is so much to look into before he gets home. For instance, one of us is in charge of house, one in charge of accessible van, one in charge of voice activated phone, one in charge of voice activated everything, and one in charge of home care. I don't think it will be a problem at all. Seriously, it is working out pretty well, especially with the resources you all have sent us, which we very much appreciate.

As always, thanks so much.

Jamie's plea for help

First Essay Assignment. Any Ideas?

Write about how quality has entered your life and the effect that this has had. You may choose one long narrative example or many shorter ones. Since the notion of quality is often subjective or relative, it would perhaps be useful to frame your narratives by opening and closing sections where your philosophical views, definitions, attitudes can be presented.

Sorry, just kind of confused?!

My response

Well, quality is subjective but I would think you could use Trenton's accident. Although it is not an altogether positive quality it doesn't have to be a negative quality. For instance, your views before the accident were possibly seeing someone in a wheelchair and feeling bad or you had empathy for them, but not until you actually experienced this with your brother did you truly understand what it means to be a quadriplegic. Explain how it has changed your life as well as Trenton's but the positive is you are aware of others' plights and you, as well as your family, are now proactive in promoting stem cell research as well as how difficult it is to live in society as a quad. We think we are a wheelchair accessible society, but think of all the places you go that most quads cannot. Another positive is it has brought friends and family closer. Love you.

I am not quite sure why I thought the following paper was going to save you. Honestly, it is a bit confusing. I can't remember what grade you got on this paper, but you may have gotten a sympathy grade!

Subject line was "Save your Ass Document"

The quality of life for everyone is different. Quality is a personal trait, a character reflecting that person. The quality of life has different standards and characteristics for each person to live by. Quality can be altered due to life altering experiences and whether we view them as a positive or negative. My quality of life has changed significantly in the past few months and has altered the lives of myself, my family, and others forever.

On June 26, 2005, my twenty-four-year old brother was celebrating his birthday at the Lake of the Ozarks with a group of friends, not knowing that this trip would change his life as well as the lives of others forever. Trenton, my brother, dove into a swimming pool and suffered a severe C4/C5 spinal cord injury. He was life flighted to a hospital in Springfield, Missouri where he spent the next four weeks in their 3rd floor ICU. He is paralyzed from the shoulders down. He was breathing with the help of a ventilator, the tubes initially in his mouth, then later a tracheotomy was inserted in his throat and he received nutrition through a tube inserted in his stomach. Due to the drugs he was taking and the trauma of the accident, Trenton has no recollection of the accident or his stay in Springfield. After the four weeks he was transferred to Craig Hospital, a premiere hospital dedicated to Spinal Cord Rehabilitation and Traumatic Brain Injuries, in Denver, Colorado. Currently Trenton is undergoing daily physical therapy classes, occupational therapy classes, as well as attending special outings with other patients. His projected time to return to Kansas City, our home, is the end of October.

Quality is subjective. As in this case, the quality of life has changed dramatically and although it would not be considered a positive it does not have to be a negative. The saying goes, "you are not given more than you can handle" but no one is prepared to handle such a life altering challenge. Because of this, you are forced to see the positive of a very negative situation. The positives you focus on are that my brother is still here and he has become an inspiration not only to me but to many others. Trenton has been the force for all of us to be able to focus on these positives. For instance, every night when I talk to him he is still my "big brother," insisting that I study, go to class, and try not to party too much. His body may be broken but mentally he is strong, determined and focused on his goals to succeed in improving his quality of life. His spirit is unwavering. He wants me to have the college experience he had. He always says, "It's the best time of your life!" He is an inspiration to all of us and because of this, our perception of quality of life has altered. I look at life differently. I try to think before I act. Not wearing my seatbelt, getting in a car with a drunk driver, and driving too fast are all actions that can ultimately change your quality of life within a split second. His life changed forever because of a meaningless dive into a shallow pool. I know right from wrong and I know good from bad. I know the choices I need to make to accomplish what I want to do.

This accident left my family and me with many questions. Why did this happen to us? Why did it happen to him? Why does it have to happen to anyone? Unfortunately, those questions cannot be answered. Not only is this accident mentally and emotionally draining, it is also financially draining. Today, my family is struggling to find a handicapped accessible home, a van, and a 24 hour caregiver for my brother. My family and I look at life completely different now. We are now proactive in promoting stem cell research; aware of others and their plight, and realizing how difficult it is to live in a society as a quadriplegic. I used to see someone in a wheelchair and feel empathy for them but now I truly understand how hard it is to live as a paraplegic or a quadriplegic. We think we are a wheelchair accessible society, but in fact our society in not very wheelchair friendly. Most homes are not accessible for wheelchairs.

My quality of life has changed significantly in the past few months and has altered the lives of myself, my family, and others forever. Although, our quality of life has changed, it is neither for the positive or negative but rather how we perceive our life today and how we choose to live our life tomorrow. Trenton is alive and we are thankful for this every day. He has been inspiring and he will continue to give words of wisdom and advice to encourage others. He is going to continue to give love and support to me and everything I do. He is going to BELIEVE in me just like everybody else BELIEVES in him.

Email from Faith (friend of mine)

Ryan has this idea that he would like to take Trenton on Tuesdays to the YMCA when they have one-on-one swimming fun/therapy in the water. Do you know if this would be something Trenton would be able to do or like to do? Ryan is so excited that he might be able to do this for Trenton. Ryan will go and get trained and take the required classes to help Trenton have fun or have it be a part of his care. What do you think? Ryan would do what he needs to do on his end and be all ready if it is a possibility.

Update from Me

Hi all,

Tonight's email could be a carbon copy of last night's so I hate to even send this one out. When I talked to Trenton tonight, he was lying in bed just as a precaution. A few had asked about the bed sores. When you are in one position for too long, your skin will start to break down as a result of lack of circulation to that area. This is why they do their weight shifts to get their circulation moving and they turn them in their bed at night. They can be serious but that would usually only happen with severe neglect. Trenton just has a red spot but they will then keep him off that spot to make sure it gets healed before it becomes anything serious.

He was up today for his classes but then chose to get in bed early tonight. He just said he was a little bored, but for the most part he sounded good. Again, I did the ramble thing and told him I had one more night of rambling and then I would be out there.

If there is nothing new tomorrow I will probably wait until I get out there Friday to write the next update.

My Email to Adam

Hi Adam,

Attached is the info on O'Dowd's. It starts at 6:00 pm and goes to midnight. Trenton is fine with the bed sore. They catch it early and treat it and then it is not a problem. The only time it is dangerous is if they don't see it and then it can get pretty bad. He does want to live on his own so hopefully that will work out. Chris and Sam are planning on living with him. I am going out tomorrow so I will call you sometime and let you talk to him. He enjoys talking to everyone.

I think the O'Dowd's will really be a nice event. I'm sure everyone is busy with last minute wedding plans. I am sure it is hard to be so far away from home. Hang in there and we can't wait to see you. I was going through pictures for Tyson to make a video and there were so many of you and Trenton. Of course I was a mess going through them, but what nice memories.

Email from Janis
Susan,

David is leaving for Columbia today. His mom asked where Trenton is headed to after Craig. Will he be going home? Continued outpatient therapy?

My Email to Janis
Hi Janis,

Sorry it has taken me so long to respond. You understand; just busy. I am so glad David is on his way. It was such a good feeling when we finally got Trenton to Craig. I just felt like that was the healing process for all of us. He leaves Craig towards the end of October, barring any complications, which no one foresees. He will do therapy but a lot of it on his own and I'm sure we will have some sort of outpatient therapy. To be honest, there are so many essentials we have to think of first, I haven't gotten to therapy yet. Amazingly, Trenton wants to try to live on his own with roommates and of course we will be there a lot, plus some nursing care. Again, we have to make some quick decisions.

Give David's mom my best and please keep me posted on David's progress, which I am sure will be leaps and bounds once he gets to rehab. You all are always in my thoughts and prayers and get the "bitchy" girlfriends out of the picture. Like we have time to deal with that also!

Email from Judy (neighbor and friend of mine)

Dear Susan:

I just recently started getting your emails from Jeff. You have done an amazing job of keeping friends abreast of Trenton's daily progress. I must admit that tears generally come as I read the challenges and progress that Trenton has made over the last several weeks. You are both AWESOME! We have had Trenton on our prayer list at church and several members of the congregation have asked me how Trenton is doing. We will certainly continue those prayers as Trenton faces some major adjustments with his move back here in the near future.

I must say I feel very guilty as a friend for not contacting you sooner but there is not a day that I have missed saying a prayer for Trenton and your whole family. I did run into Jane at Kohl's this weekend and heard about the house for Trenton. Sewers are rather important, so guess we better hope progress is made there in a rapid manner.

We do have a new member to our family. Sadly, we had to put Spud to sleep in early August but three weeks ago Jay and John showed up at home with a three month old Lab puppy that is "red." His name is Gus and he is really adorable and he is going to be "really" big! Jay certainly knows how to pick them! You must see him when you have a chance. Well, since I'm at work, I best get back to work. Take care and give my greetings to Trenton as well.

Email from Denise

Hey Susan,

Last week wasn't that great but this week is better. Brian is flying to Chicago and meeting up with three of his frat brothers to see the Cubs vs Cardinals game at Wrigley. He has always been a Cubbies fan. So, he has something to look forward to, which is a good thing.

He has the second round of chemo starting next Monday. He tolerated the first round so I don't expect any surprises. His blood tests were good after the first round and that was nice news. I'm just praying this shit works. It is $8,000 for 5 days' worth of pills . . . it has to be good, right?!

I just need to go to Houston and hear that the residual tumor is shrinking, etc. Of course, the best thing to hear is it's gone, but I don't think it has been enough time or doses.

I know you will be so glad to get Trenton back to KC. Do you need help moving stuff from his apt to his new house? I have the Explorer if you need to borrow it.

UMKC is fine. I drive him every day and then find some way to entertain myself while he is at class. We leave around 9:00 am and get home around 2:30 pm. If seizure free (and there is no reason to think otherwise) he will be driving by Halloween.

Email from Ryan (friend who is a physical therapist)
Susan and Trenton,

I have talked to some of my professors to get some ideas for when Trenton gets back to KC! I have been told that the ALS association is very helpful and you can purchase a wheelchair accessible van through this organization. They can point you to resources for van purchase and adaptations for driving and moving the wheelchair.

There is a SCI support group based at Rehab Institute that might be able to assist in the transition back home and other future needs. There is also a vocational rehab program there to assist with planning for the future.

The seating clinics here at KU and at MidAmerican partner with local vendors. It would be most beneficial to have this team approach that can access needs, understand equipment options and negotiate funding. I have been told that Craig has a great seating clinic so this may not be necessary.

I hope this helps out in any way. Let me know if I can do anything else. Can't wait to hang out you with soon Trenton. GO CHIEFS!

September 14 Update from Me
Hello,

Just a quick update. I have had some questions as to whether Trenton will be able to make the O'Dowd's event. Unfortunately, he will not, but I am taping him this weekend and Tyson (my son-in-law) is putting it into a video that will be running during the event. It is the best we can do but Tyson is a genius when it comes to this stuff and he puts together awesome videos. (No pressure Tyson.)

Trenton is scheduled, barring no complications, to come home around October 26th. We will have another family conference Tuesday, September 27th and I am sure we will find out more then.

I talked to him a few minutes ago and he was in his chair watching TV. He is looking forward to this weekend. I didn't talk to him for very long as he had the TV up so loud I couldn't hear him so I just acted like I knew what he saying. He was totally convinced.

Tomorrow's update will be live, since I will be out there.

September 15, Friday, Update from Me

Hi all,

We are out here with Trenton and he is doing really well. Derek and Jill, Tessa, Lexi and Scott got here about midnight last night and Ric 2 and I got here about 1:00. Trenton is now tube free with the latest being his feeding tube being removed. Today he went down for a neck X-ray to see if he can get the brace off. Chuck and Kristi are coming in tonight. Trenton was told today that he has to change rooms as there is someone coming in who needs to be directly across from the nurse's station, so he will move across the hall. It is still a private room but if you could see all the stuff we have, it will take a while to get him moved. We are just sitting here talking about his first month stay in Springfield. He remembers nothing of it. His first recollection is getting on the plane to come out to Denver.

The weather is beautiful here and they had a woman playing the saxophone so we went out to listen to her for a while. They had Kool-Aid and some appetizers.

He is waiting to get a shower and then wants to get back in his chair so he can visit and watch TV with everyone. Tomorrow he wants to cook out and then, of course, the Chiefs play Sunday night.

Email from Adam

That is too bad Trenton can't make it to the O'Dowd's event.

How is his voice, is it strong or weak? Tell him I said hi and I miss him a lot. I want to send him a card but don't know if I should buy a sympathetic one or a funny one. What are other people doing? Sometimes I just don't know what to do to show sympathy or to try and shed some light on the situation, so I have just been sitting back and praying for him. I really miss him and hope he is doing well (do I annoy you with all my email replies?) I am going skydiving this weekend, so cross your fingers and hope the parachute opens. Has Trenton been able to move his arms yet, is the feeling in his chest getting better? Are his spirits up or is he depressed? Tell him he means so much to me and has been my oldest friend I have ever had. He was my very first friend.

All right, I have rambled too much, I need to get to bed. Love you guys' lots. Tell Trenton GO CHIEFS, and that we are going to beat the Raiders asses this weekend. I hate the Raiders. Did he hear about Larry Johnson and that he was arrested on Monday for beating his girlfriend? I don't understand these NFL guys.

September 19, Tuesday, Update from Me

Hi all,

Trenton had a good weekend with his friends. A lot of football was watched and we had BBQ Saturday night. The weather was so great. Friday the hospital told us he was going to have to move to another room as there was someone who needed to be by the nurse's station. It was great since there were so many people here so we packed him up and moved him down the hall and the girls had everything back on the walls within an hour.

He is supposed to be weaning from his collar but the nurse came in and said it really was up to him if he wanted to put it back on and Trenton said he wanted it off for good. He looks good. I taped a bit of him for Thursday night and his room to show all the posters and pictures he has received.

September 20, Wednesday, Update from Me

Hello,

It is never easy for any of us to leave Trenton and today was no exception. The difference today was he was sound asleep so I didn't wake him when I left. He was exhausted last night and fell asleep by 7:30 and was still asleep when I tried to call him before we got on the plane at 10:00 this morning. I have no idea why he was so tired but yesterday in OT the therapist had told him he may be more tired the first few days his neck brace is off. She was also telling him his neck muscles were pretty strong and for his type of injury this was great as he can do so much with his neck. For example, she showed me a stick with 2 prongs at the end and when placed in your mouth you can turn pages of a book. She said Trenton was able to do this the first time he tried, which was good, considering his injury. I remember when we were in Springfield and the admissions lady from Craig came to talk with us. She told us that Trenton would be able to do more things than he cannot when he returned home from Craig. We are doing our best to believe this.

I am amazed each time I go out there with Trenton's attitude. I was telling him of a paper that Jamie had to do about "quality of life." Of course she used Trenton's accident as an example and how quality of life had a lot to do with your perception. I told him she wrote that although his experience was not a positive it didn't have to be a totally negative one. To which he replied that there was nothing positive about this but you have to move on and not dwell on the "what ifs". I know there are times he thinks about the "what ifs" as we all do, but I am so impressed that he is doing his best not to dwell on them and concentrating instead on working as hard as he can to improve his situation. They say at Craig there are small miracles every day. The problem is, every patient there is praying for the big one.

I will probably do updates every other day or so because there is just not as much to write on a day-to-day basis now that he is tube free and brace free. Everyone has been so wonderful and I know I have said this before but it is worth saying again; we could not and cannot do this without you.

Email from Ryan (physical therapist)
Trenton,
Hey buddy, I got great news. I applied for a scholarship in

which our department is sponsoring one student to attend the Physical Therapy National Student Conclave in Denver. I will be out there the weekend of October 21st. I believe that is your last week at Craig so hopefully it will work out for me to see you. I am very intrigued to see the hospital and especially your room...it sounds like you pimped it out. I am sure that I have a busy schedule of meeting (I only applied for it so I could skip school and, really, to see you), but I will do my best to get out of some of them. The only downfall is that I am required to present my experience back to the faculty and students. Anyways, I will definitely find time for us to catch up. Talk to you soon.

PS--The Chiefs didn't look great on Sunday but at least we pulled out the win. The commentators were so annoying. All they talked about was how great Randy Moss is. It showed how much we need Roaf back in the offense.

Email from Trevor (friend of yours from high school)

Hi there. I am glad to hear that Trenton is doing so well. I wish him the best and think about him every day. I can't wait till he gets home so that I can visit. If you need anything when it comes time for him to come home, just let me know. I would be glad to help move or help him get settled in. Whatever you need, I will see what I can do for you. I wish that I knew more about the voice activated stuff for him, but I really don't, but I am keeping my eyes and ears open for you.

But I had a question to ask you. I know that Rick is affiliated with the new O'Dowd's, but I wasn't sure how. My question is, I was wondering if they needed any help with bartenders and/or waitresses. My fiancé had been waiting tables for a long time for Outback Steakhouse in Lee's Summit, but doesn't so much want to drive out there all the time. I wasn't sure if they were fully staffed or if they were still in need of help. She would be interested if they are.

Well I look forward to seeing you all on Thursday. Talk to you later. And thanks for the updates.

Email from Janis

Suzi,

David's mom has set up a link for David. If you are interested you register and sign in and then it will ask you for patient information and then direct you to his page. David's mom put a few photos up yesterday. Do you have a similar page for Trenton?

Email response to Janis

Hi Janis,

I just got it to work and David looks wonderful. I can't believe the difference. We certainly have been through a lot haven't we? I am so happy that David is in a good place and is now on his road to recovery.

The O'Dowd's Event and scrambling to get you ready to come home.

September 25, Monday, Update from Me

Hello,

I am one of these people who writes thank yous for thank yous. You know, thank you for writing me a thank you. I'm not really quite that bad but close, so you can imagine what the O'Dowd's event did to me. We are all extremely appreciative for the support the other night. Although we wish the get together had been for a different reason, we sincerely hope that you enjoyed yourself. The event was a huge success because of all of you. Rick, Cathy, Jane, and Ashley were instrumental in organizing the event. Tyson did a great job with the video and we appreciate Tim (Rick's brother) auctioneering for us. We also greatly appreciate Larry and Judy, Betty, Emily, Martha, Tom and Marcy, Jim and Julie for manning the door. Of course, we appreciate the management of O'Dowd's for allowing us to have the event. Jim was so thoughtful to come and take pictures. Tangela did an awesome job with the marketing of the event. It was very nice of Steve and his wife Debbie to come and speak. He had just gotten back into town and was most gracious to say a few inspirational words. Ok, you can probably see where this is going. By the end of this update I could and should thank each of you individually.

We all wanted so much to get around and talk to every one of you and by going through the index cards, I see that I missed so many of you.

During the event, I called Trenton and was telling him about it. He was concerned about people waiting to get on the deck and O'Dowd's running out of Bud Light and Miller Light. He also wanted me to get everyone's name so he could write thank yous.

This coming from a kid I used to have to stand over, put a pen in his hand and say "write." Suffice it to say, he is very touched by the overwhelming support.

Trenton is doing well and looking forward to the Broncos/Chiefs game. Rick is going out today and I am going out Monday. We have our family conference Tuesday and I am hoping they will give us a definite date for his homecoming.

Some of you have mentioned you wanted a t-shirt and didn't get one. Ashley has them and you can call her to let her know what size you would like.

It has been three months since the accident, although it seems so much longer. Everyone's faith is tested at some point and you do what you have to do but it certainly helps to have the support of family and friends. Thanks again to all of you for a fun and successful event.

The O'Dowd's event was amazing. So many people came to offer their support. Your dad spoke and Tyson had made a video of you that was played throughout the night. Honestly, I could not believe the crowd. It was truly amazing.

Email from Keri (friend of yours)
Susan,

It was so nice to finally meet you in person Thursday night. The event was incredible, and it just shows how many people pray for Trenton. I wanted to let you know a couple of things that I wanted to share with you Thursday night, but of course it was such a busy night for you and your family. Barry (not sure on the spelling) is a great guy that I went to college with at SMS and we worked at the same bar. It's very odd that he was in a shallow diving accident like Trenton. When I reflect back with working with Barry it's so weird how Trenton and he are so alike in so many ways. They both have incredible personalities that people are instantly drawn to. They are both frat guys that love to go out and be social (which I know Barry still does because I've seen him out at the Granfaloon). I was excited to hear that Trenton would be in contact with Barry because I think the two of them have much in common.

I also wanted to let you know that my husband and I are having another baby in April, and because of Trenton we are going to save the cord which contains stem cells. We debated with our last baby, but Trenton's situation has made the decision very easy. Again, it was wonderful to meet you and we will continue to pray for Trenton and your family!

Email from Judy (friend of our family)
Susan,

Larry and I loved working at the door. Please let us help whenever we can. What an inspirational evening, so many people showing their love for Trenton and his family. Most people can only count their friends on one hand. Trenton is definitely a remarkable young man. Take care. We will see you in Colorado in a week. Give our best to Trenton! Love, Judy

Email from Susie (friend of mine)
Susan,

I just wanted to tell you how impressed we were with the turnout for Trenton's fundraiser. You all did a great job in organizing! You all have such great friends! I am with you, I am sorry for the reason for the event, but I did have a great time, so many people to see and talk to!

I was just wondering how much $$ you were able to raise? Is Trenton going to be able to use all the $$ for his care?

Even though the game was so horrible last night, I hope Trenton enjoyed the outing!

September 27, Wednesday, Update from Me
Hi all,

You can imagine all the grief Trenton is getting because of the Chief's poor performance last night. His comebacks have been, "I believe both teams are 2 and 1" and "Broncos still have to play at

Arrowhead this year." In spite of the turnout, they had a great time. Trenton wore his Derrick Thomas jersey and he loaned his other jersey to a fellow Chief's fan who went also. John was able to get them field passes before the game to watch the Bronco's warm up. All in all, they had a great time. Trenton thought their stadium was awesome but the fans were not as loud as the Chiefs.

We had our conference today. Dr. Chi was very positive regarding Trenton's progress and his attitude. He reiterated Trenton's agenda, which was first to get off the vent, next remove the trach and to then to start eating. Dr. Chi felt he had done all this in record time. Mary, his physical therapist, said his PT was going well and Donna, his occupational therapist, said that once Trenton made up his mind, he did, in fact, learn to drive his wheelchair in a day, just like he said he would. To which I said "show off" and she said "exactly." His projected release date is October 28th but we are not to make plane arrangements quite yet, just in case there is a setback with equipment coming in, etc. The other good news is they (Craig Hospital) make all the arrangements. We make sure he has a place to live and a van and they order all equipment and help with home care. Our job is to learn how to care for Trenton in every aspect and become educated on complications which can occur with spinal cord injuries. We will have one more conference the week of the 26th to finalize everything for his release.

As we were walking through the hospital today, Trenton was acknowledging everyone. We all feel bad when no one is with him, which isn't often, but maybe it has done him some good to socialize, which is what Trenton does best. He has his "Hi I wanna lei ya" Hawaiian t-shirt on so he showed it to Layton. Layton said he was usually a little more discreet with his pickup lines. Again, we want to thank you all for the success of O'Dowd's.

I received an email at this time that David had died. I didn't want to put the actual email in this. It was truly heartbreaking and certainly difficult to understand. I am unsure as to what happened to this young man. He had been doing very well.

Email from Nathan

Hello,

Well, I hope you had more fun at the game then I did watching it. Here is the final information on the concert. It is Friday, October 14th. Tickets at the door are going to be $10. They will be $7 if bought before. It starts at 8 pm. I need your address so that I can send you 4 tickets. Or I guess however many family members you have coming up.

Derick said he would talk for a little bit. If you would want to talk with him that would be awesome. Just something about what happened, why we are doing this, and what it all means. Stuff like that. T-shirts will be on sale for $10. How many people do you think from Kansas City will be coming up?

I think that is about it....Let me know if there is anything else you need or want or whatever. I couldn't make it to the O'Dowd's event because I had a test the next morning, but I hear it was a huge success. That's awesome!

Email from Ashley

How would October 20th through the 24th be for me coming out? Will you be there this weekend or not? Let me know so I can buy my ticket. Let me know what time your flight gets in tomorrow so I can pick you up, I really don't mind. I am overtime on Friday so they might cancel me anyways and I am only there till 3 if I do have to work. Love you. Tell Trenton hi.

My response to Ashley

I am here the 17th - 20th so that would work out perfectly. I will buy your ticket. Just tell me how much it is. Jamie knows about Sunday. She always finds out the secrets.

I get in at 9:30 tomorrow night on Frontier.

Thanks and love you. We just watched Hostage with Bruce Willis, last night I Robots or whatever.

Email from Adam

I think I am going to get him the shirt, "Show me your boobs and

I will pop a wheelie." I think he will like that one the most. Don't you? I just wanna make sure I got the right address before I buy it and send it.

I wrote you already once tonight about how I found this website of funny handicap shirts. I put the link on my favorites. Check them out and see if you think Trenton would like the shirts or not. You can browse the site, but I just wanted to put my favorite shirt links on there. I think Trenton would like these a lot, but not for sure.

October 3, Tuesday, Update from Me

Hello,

Trenton is doing well, bored, but doing well. I left last Thursday with him in his OT class and he and Donna, his therapist, were on the computer making the football picks for the weekend. Donna was showing me different options Trenton could use when he gets home. He could have a work station with magnetic sticks. He then could get a stick with his mouth and use it to turn pages in a book or one could be used to write with and another to type with on the computer. Each stick would go back onto its magnetic base so he wouldn't need anyone to help him. It is not Trenton's favorite means of functioning but he does pretty well with it and it could certainly work for a while.

When he leaves October 28th, his stay will have been three months, which is the minimum most people stay. Some stay as long as a year, depending on complications, etc. We are very lucky that his stay and progress have gone so well. I think Trenton (although it will be somewhat of an adjustment when he does come home) would go crazy if he had to stay much longer. Trust me, the staff is wonderful but it is a very monotonous life.

He did have a Bronco party, not by his choice, but the nurses all congregated in his room yesterday to watch the game. He also had a surprise visitor this morning-Randy Grodishar, an ex-Bronco player. The nurses were not happy with him when they found out and Trenton didn't call them to let them know he was here. A huge thanks to Fred and Linda for setting this up. I think he got quite a kick out of it. He left him a signed picture and a Bronco jersey, which he wants to get framed. The staff thinks he is pretty spoiled, thanks to all of you.

October 6, Friday, Update from Me

I left Trenton tonight knowing that Jamie was flying in to surprise him. She had not seen him since August; therefore she had not seen him vent-free, trach-free, eating and talking. Trust me, she needed to see him. I had a hard time keeping it a secret but she arrived about 9:30 and he was thrilled.

Today I learned how to transport Trenton in his manual chair up and down stairs and up and down curbs. It is not my favorite thing to do as these chairs are heavy and difficult to maneuver. I am sure Trenton was nervous also but he was a real trooper and didn't say a word when I was jerking him all over the place. Because his re-entry class was cancelled, we visited with Leighton, his father, and Danny and his family. I am constantly amazed by their stories and the magnitude of the injuries and how it has changed their lives. Leighton had been in a Hawaii hospital for eight months before being transferred to Craig. By the time he left the hospital his bill was close to a million dollars. The hospital had no idea what to do with his injury and basically kept him alive. Leighton said he just laid in bed for those eight months and watched TV. His injury is a C2/3 but he has some finger movement in his left hand and is vent free. Danny went over a cliff in his car and broke nearly his entire spinal column and was told he would never walk again and is walking some now. You never hear them complain; they talk about what they hope to accomplish in the future and what type of work they will be doing when they get home.

We then went to OT and they hooked Trenton up with a system in which he is able to sip and puff his fan, lights, TV and DVD on and off. It is remarkable what you can do with a straw-like device. Leighton was talking about how much we take for granted. He commented that he wished he could just scratch his face and brush his teeth. Everyone agreed, but they also said they believed they would be able to someday.

Jamie was having a rough time. It was her first year of college and she was balancing sorority with school work and, on top of all that, she was thinking of you and wishing she could see you more. I had mentioned it was difficult for me to go out and do normal things and have fun because I was always thinking of you. I know Jamie and Ashley were feeling this way as well. I was taking Jamie back to school one weekend and had to pull over due to her anxiety because it was making her sick. I really felt she needed some professional help so she saw Dr. K and got something for it. I also had to make sure I was able to be available for those important times in their lives. We all knew this was a life change and not anything that was going to resolve soon, so I had to learn to balance my time.

Email from Adam

Hey Susan,

I ordered Trenton the shirt, "Show me your boobs and I will pop a wheelie." I hope he likes it and I got an email today that it got out in the mail by the company and he should be getting it either tomorrow or Monday. Just to let you know.

Glad he is doing well. I am trying to call him every couple of days now to talk.

October 8, Sunday, Update from Me

Hi,

Judy and Larry came in Monday night. Judy's cousin lives here but they have stopped by every day to see Trenton. It really has been nice to have them here. Since they drove, they are also going to take a lot of Trenton's things back with them. Trenton is getting a little nervous with all his valuable signed footballs, cleats and jerseys here. His room looks a little bare but it is worth it to not have to drive back here to get it all home. Since it was a Monday night, Judy and Larry got to see the Newfoundlands. Lucy, who is also a show dog, was doing all sorts of tricks for them. They really are the most amazing dogs.

Trenton is busy in all his classes getting ready to check out of here. In PT we are discussing the different types of beds available which he needs to make a decision on soon so he will have one when he gets home. Today in OT they went over some different choices for computer software and voice activated phones, etc. He also started his re-entry classes. There are 18 in this class, which means lots of patients are going home soon. They discuss getting back into the workforce or school, whichever applies. Everyone took turns telling what they used to do and whether they thought they could go back to what they had been doing. There were teachers, a composer, students, etc. Layton from Hawaii used to be a fisherman and also did a little carpentry. He said carpentry was boring so he thought he would just watch his grass grow. The guy who led the class today has a yellow lab who is his trained lead dog. He was saying this dog is worth $15,000. I don't think Trenton will be getting one anytime soon, but what a great dog! I am trying to talk Trenton into getting a chimpanzee but he will have no part of it. Again, I keep saying this, but I give him so much credit. He is probably doing better than the rest of us, which they actually said was not uncommon. He is planning for the future and is so eager to get home.

Last night we were watching Kill Bill and his nurse and techs brought their work in and watched the movie with us. They told me when we aren't with him they are in his room a lot. In fact, they made him host a Bronco party in his room last weekend for the game.

There is still so much up in the air, but we have so much to be thankful for and even though there are days when we don't have a clue how we are getting through this and we don't want to deal with any of this and we are mad at the world (I'm being a little dramatic) we know we will get through this because we basically have no choice.

Rick had asked me to attach the following and I kept forgetting, so here it is. Thanks.

Sent on behalf of Rick Baier

As I have stated in the past I want to thank all of you for the support you have given Trenton and my family since his June 26 accident. I appreciate many of you attending our thank you event at

O'Dowd's last Thursday. We had well over 600 people attend and it allowed us to launch the Trenton R. Baier Believe Trust Fund very successfully. Over $20,000 was raised that night to support Trenton, as well as research for spinal injuries. More importantly, we were able to thank the community for their fabulous support. I have just returned from Denver last night. Trenton and I attended the Chiefs-Broncos game and through the efforts of Jon of CB Richard Ellis we were able to have field passes during the pregame. We were in the Bronco end zone and I can tell you that those Broncos were fired up. In spite of the outcome, we had a great time. Tuesday we met with all of Trenton's doctors and nurses and I am pleased to report that he has been scheduled to leave Craig Hospital October 28. Trenton is off all support systems now and is eating and talking well. He has a great attitude and is looking forward to his next stage of life. He wants his own house and we are looking at that possibility now. There will be challenges for a long time but we will still win this war. We are all so proud of Trenton and we thank you for all your prayers, donations, cards, calls and letters. I could not have picked a better career where I could have built such a strong network of true friends. Thank you!

Email from Stephanie

Hi Susan, it was good to hear from you. I guess you are in Colorado? If so, tell Trenton hi from me. I didn't send a card today, I've been kind of on a roll. In fact I told him to not worry. I swear I'm not stalking him. He's just on my mind so much and you are too. In fact, all of you are. Your family is very important to me. I feel a connection, I just do. Trenton has been part of my world for a long time and as I'm sure you have figured out, is very special to me. I just want you to know that I mean it when I say, if there is anything you might need, I will always be here to help. I'm glad to hear that he's doing well. He really is amazing. I am sure he will hit rough patches but I do believe that he will shine bright. I want you to also know that I very much admire you and how gracefully you are handling this, at least on the outside. I can only imagine as a parent how hard this is every single moment. You really are doing great! You are in my prayers every day.

OK, so anyway, give Trenton my love. I can't wait to see him. Take care of you. I am going to forward you a couple of jokes, share them with Trenton, they are kind of funny.

Email from Beau (your cousin)

Hey Susan,

Its Beau, I am in Kuwait and getting ready for my unit's trip north to Iraq. Gonna do some work there with my unit and do the job we were trained for. Other than that, not much going on here in Kuwait. Just real hot and sandy. It's ok though. They feed us like four meals a day and have decent places to sleep. Tell Trenton I said hi and that I hope things continue to get better for him. I hope to see him when I get back in a year or more. Tell everyone else hi for me too.

Email from Barbara (friend of the family)

Hi Susan

I'm sure you get tons of emails per day, but I have been wanting to let you know that we're thinking of you and your family. Denise has been sharing your emails with me and I just wanted to let you know I look forward to them every day. I hope you're keeping all of them. You may want to write a book someday. Trenton is amazing!

I know you're getting all kinds of information thrown at you, but I just wanted you to know that in the future, if Trenton wants to start thinking about vocational options, the Division of Vocational Rehabilitation is available to him. If he is interested at some point, I know some of the people in the north office and I would be happy to steer you to someone I know and trust. I know a lot of people in the vocational rehab community in KC and would be happy to help Trenton navigate the waters when he's ready.

I see where you have an interest in service dogs. There is a volunteer organization you may have heard of that trains and provides dogs for people who need them. I used to do some fundraising for them (years ago) and at one point was thinking of taking one of their dropouts from the program. They have very strict standards and after initial training, if the dog doesn't meet their standards, they discontinue training. The name of the organization is

Canine Companions for Independence.

Anyhow, I just wanted you to know we're thinking of you and if there is anything we can do, please let us know. Jerry and I were sorry we couldn't make the O'Dowd's event, but please let us know if there is anything we can do.

October 10, Tuesday, Update from Me

Hi,

Trenton and Jamie had a good weekend. They went to a Mexican party for Danny, who is to be discharged soon, and had authentic Mexican food. The rest of the weekend they watched football and visited.

Unfortunately, Trenton is not feeling well at all today and did not get out of bed. He is dehydrated and is on IV. They say nothing to worry about, but of course you do anyway, although I am sure he just has not been drinking enough fluids, which, of course, is the meaning of dehydration. Thankfully, Rick is out there with him and says Trenton feels pretty puny right now.

We have some new leads with a house and some of the other essentials. I will let you know if anything works out. I don't want to sound negative but at this point I don't want to jinx anything.

I know this is short but when I am not there it is harder to write newsy updates. Rick is just not as detail-oriented as I am, which is probably a blessing.

Email from Mary Alice (friend of mine)

Dear Susan,

I don't tell you often enough, but we're so appreciative of the updates on Trenton. He's always in our thoughts and prayers. I'm sorry he's not feeling well, and I know you worry, but he sure has lots of prayers going up for him.

I'm assuming that you're here in KC right now, by your note. Is there anything - ANYTHING - that I can do to help you? I love you and want to be of help.

Email chain with Jamie

Good Morning--

Our skit didn't make it... Oh well! Plan on me taking your ticket and sitting with you if you don't care! Have a good day! Love you lots

My reply:

Hi there,

I am sorry your skit did not win, maybe your house will win best house decorations. Julie says that the Farmhouse usually wins.

I would be honored to have you sit with me at the Chiefs game; it is supposed to be a lovely day! Have a great one.

Love you and miss you!

Email from Nathan

Hi,

Well, it's finally here. The concert on this Friday. Here is the schedule for how it should all go down.

Schedule for Friday...

4:00-SF LOAD IN
4:30-SF SOUND CHECK
6:00-SLANG 5 LOAD IN
6:30-SLANG 5 SOUND CHECK
7:00-JOEY/ NATHAN/ SUSAN RUN THRU
7:30-DOORS OPEN- EVERYONE OFF STAGE
8:00-SHOW STARTS
8:15-SLANG 5 ON STAGE
9:00-SUSAN ON STAGE
9:10/15- SF ON STAGE
11:00 CLEAN UP

If you could let me know if you are staying overnight or not and where, that would be great. Also, if you could call me and let me know when you get into town that would help also.

Joey and I are going to introduce the bands and you. We are just acting like MCs. I am going to thank everyone who is coming out and just give some basic facts off of the Christopher Reeve's website. Whatever you want to talk about is fine. How is Trenton doing? Is he is coming back home, what will happen, etc. Thank you very much for helping with that. The show is going to be amazing. It wouldn't be without your help. So again, thank you.

October 12, Thursday, Update from Me

I really have nothing to tell you except that Trenton is feeling better. He is still on IV fluids but he did get up and go to his classes today. The problem is, he is just not drinking enough, so until he does, he will have to be supplemented. I only talked to him briefly yesterday and he did sound better. I don't think this will have any impact on his coming home the 28th but I guess if he doesn't improve on his fluid intake, it could.

I go back out the 17th so I will have a little more information. Hopefully, the Chiefs will have a great game Sunday and Trenton will have done well in his fantasy football.

I probably won't write again until Monday unless something comes up so have a great weekend a little early.

Email from Michelle (friend of Trenton's)

Susan,

This is Michelle and I just have a quick question for you. I have been sending Trenton cards and I just realized that I have sent the last three or four and forgotten to put Ste. 230 on them. I just wanted to make sure they were still getting to him. Also, I was not sure if he could talk on the phone or if I e-mailed to him if he could read it. I was just wondering because I would love to be able to talk to him more than just through the cards. I think about all of you every day and I miss Trenton so much. I cannot wait until he is home so I can see him all the time. I love you all very much.

My Email to Michelle

Hi Michelle,

How is San Diego? Do you love it? The weather is sure perfect. Trenton is not in room 230 anymore as they needed that room for a man who needed to be right across from the nurse's station, so he is in room 224. It doesn't matter. If you put his name, it will get to him. You can also email him to my email and he just wheels up to the computer to read it. He loves for people to call him also. Just call the front desk and ask for Trenton and they will run down and put it on speaker phone so he can talk. He really enjoys talking to everyone and everyone is always so amazed how good he sounds.

We think we may have a place for him to live, just hope it works out. I hope you are having a good time and keep in touch. Trenton is supposed to come home the 28th and I thought when I found out the time he would arrive I would let everyone know and whoever could meet him at the airport.

October 13, Friday, Update from Me

Well I told you I would not write again until Monday unless I had something exciting to tell you and I have good news. We have a place for Trenton to live with Chris and Sam. It is a villa, brand new, just off Oak Street behind Oak Park High School. We can move him October 27th, which is perfect. Trenton is excited but is concerned because it only has two bedrooms and not a huge yard for his huge dog, Willy. Not to worry, the basement is huge and I am calling out to anyone and everyone, if you have any ability to help us get a third bedroom ready for them. And it has a great front yard so I am sure Willy will have plenty of romping room. Trenton is feeling great again and really is excited to have a place to live. So if you want to help, please let me know. I really don't think it will take too much. Thanks, I just had to share the good news.

October 15, Sunday, Update from Me

Me again,

*Last night Rick, Ashley, Tyson, Ric 2, Karen and I attended a Benefit for Baier at Northwest Missouri State University organized by Nathan, who is a Sig Ep and friend of Trenton's. There were two bands which performed, **Slang 5** and **The Sound and the Fury**. We were all so impressed. Nathan did an amazing job of organizing this event. I had not met Nathan before last night but felt like I knew him through all our emailing back and forth. He is great and we appreciate what he did for Trenton and the Christopher Reeve Foundation so much. The Sig Ep house has decided to donate proceeds from their philanthropic projects to the Christopher Reeve*

Foundation and the Trenton R. Baier Trust Fund. We cannot thank Nathan, the Sig Ep house and the bands enough for putting on this event.

Thanks also to all who responded willing to help with the villa and the move. Rick will close on it October 24th and at that point I believe we can start moving him in. They are working on it this weekend, modifying the bathroom and finishing things up. Of course, my job was to make sure he had a bed and because of a little mix up, he may not have one. You would think I could get a bed ordered in time. Anyway, I'm sure it will all work out. I go out Monday and will find out what time he comes in on Friday the 28th. Again, thanks for offering to help and I will keep you posted on when we can start.

Thanks again to Nathan for last night.

Email from Adam

Hey Susan

Called Trenton yesterday and he said that he really liked the shirt. I hope he does, I know he says he does, but just wanna make sure. Has he said anything to you? I know the shirt is a little harsh, but I think it is right up Trenton's alley with his humor. Did he like it? That's really it, I think he sounds great and I am jealous of how well his fantasy football team is doing because mine isn't doing that well.

October 17, Tuesday, My response to Adam

Hi Adam,

Sorry I am just now getting back with you. Had a very busy weekend. I just got into Trenton's room and he has the t-shirt you sent him on, so he likes it very much. Thank you. He seems a little down but maybe just tired. Anyway, he always seems this way when I get out here. Thanks again for the shirt and I will let you know what time he comes in on the 28th. Hope all is well with you.

My email to Rick Baier regarding Trenton coming home

I talked to Stephanie just now and they will let us know tomorrow if Trenton will be coming home the 28th. She just wants to check with Dr. Chi. She will then make reservations for us to bring him home, probably on United leaving at 10:25 in the morning. Our conference next week is the 27th @ 3:00 pm. I will probably come out the 25th but will not rent a car and she does not want you to rent a car either because she said it will take both of us to help in the van getting him out to the airport. You will need to make sure the van you are using to pick up Trenton at the airport can hold both chairs unless the electric folds up; then it won't be a problem. Let me know if you have any questions.

Email from Adam

I am really glad Trenton was wearing the shirt. That makes me feel good. I have bad news on the 28th. I am not going to be able to make it back for his homecoming. I told Trenton this sometime last week, but I don't know if he can hear me well when I call. I don't know if it is my cell phone connection or what it is. Anyway, that is the weekend my company is going to send me to the territory that they are going to assign me to. So far I believe it is going to Sacramento and they are going to fly us out on the 26th and I won't get back until that Sunday, which is the 30th. I am pretty upset that I can't make it back for Trenton's homecoming. I am going to try and come back that following weekend. I really wanna see him and talk to him. I bet he is excited to come back.

My email to Adam

Don't worry about that weekend. Hope you have a good trip. Sacramento would be a good place to move to. Whenever you get home just look him up. He is going to the Pitt State/NWMSU game on the 29th and is looking forward to it. Take care of yourself and he understands.

Update from Me

Hello,

I am back in Colorado and I was thinking today as I got on the airplane that we have one more trip to make out here and that will be to bring Trenton home. We are all anxious but none more so than Trenton. I talked to the social worker today and we will finalize his flight tomorrow for the 28th but Trenton has put in his request for the first flight out. Craig is terrific and the people are wonderful but it is time to bring him home. I showed him the pictures of the house that Ashley had taken and he is excited to have a place of his own. He is also planning on going to the NWMSU/Pitt State game on the 29th and wants to see everyone!

Good news with the bed. They think it will be delivered maybe a little early and I actually saved us $500, although I'm not sure how, so it was a good mess up.

I wore the t-shirt we got from the Sig Ep benefit and he thought they were great. He really has an amazing attitude but he obviously has his moments. I know this weekend was hard for him; my nephew got married and Trenton was supposed to be in the wedding. He really didn't want to talk about it much.

I will let you know what reservations we make tomorrow. Thanks.

We are coming home, ready or not

October 19, Thursday, Update from Me

Hi,

I finally got the okay to make plane reservations today for the 28th. His wheelchair came in but the module was not working on it, which is amazing considering it cost $15,000, so "the team" was not sure if they would let him go home. I think we all would have lost it but today Donna with PT told us she thought it would be ok. I was on the phone as soon as we got back to the room with the travel agency and within 1/2 hour I had the tickets in hand. We arrive on Friday, the 28th, United Flight #1246 at 12:45pm. If anyone would like to meet him at the airport, I think he would love it.

We started the day with recreational therapy. In this class, he was given lots of information on recreational activities he would be able to do. Craig has invented a sip and puff fishing pole but can't get anyone to make them. Trenton, Layton, Jerry and even Goldie were very interested in this. Fortunately for us, they give you the schematics for making it and maybe we will find an engineer one day who can figure it out and make him one. I love these classes because we all end up chatting about where everyone is from, how they injured themselves and when their release date is. Jerry is 54 years old and he has a C3 injury incomplete. His wife was telling me that he had gotten up during the night to use the restroom, slipped and fell on his face and broke his neck. It was then they found out he had a degenerative bone disease which causes his bones to break more easily. Everyone is being released within two weeks of each other. Of course everyone is excited to get out of here but they also talked about how Craig is safe with everything wheelchair accessible. While everyone is pretty much in the same boat, there are still concerns as to how different the real world will be to them

now. Trenton mentioned he hasn't been sleeping too well anticipating
coming home. He is still planning on the Northwest Missouri State
University/Pitt State game on the 29th.

As I am writing this Trenton is trying to take a nap but there are
so many people in and out of his room anymore, he does not get to
rest much. He sits under this light with his Chiefs blanket because he
is always freezing. There is a guy here who looks like ET because he
always has a blanket covering him and one over his head.

I look back on these last four months and know that we would all
give anything if the accident had not happened, but it did, and
hopefully we have and will make the best of it. I know Trenton
has and he would tell you that he has met some wonderful people
and that friendships have grown. He would also tell you that he
would relive June 26th and change the outcome if he could.

I leave tomorrow morning and meet Ashley in the airport to give
her the rental car and she will stay through the weekend. Thanks to
everyone offering to help with the house. We will get Trenton settled
and then start on the basement. I know I get a little redundant and
sometimes a little sappy but all of us would say the same as Trenton;
we have met some wonderful people and friendships have grown.

Email from Adam

We have weekly speakers at our company that put on
presentations about insurance type matters. This past Tuesday my
neighbor had to give one and he gave it on disability insurance. He
used Trenton's story in his speech just to show how life can change
tremendously. He also found a resource and a nice lady from Ohio
that is a paraplegic. He found her while he was researching. She
can help give advice, I took from the presentation, on disability
insurance and what might be the best way. I shot her an email, and
haven't replied back to her. But if you guys are at all interested in
her or her story or her resources, you can find her on the net. Her
name is Rosemarie. She has her own website. If she can't help you
with any insurance I am sure she could be a motivational friend for
Trenton. She has accomplished a lot since her accident and could
share her story with Trenton, possibly, or just help. (I don't know),
but I thought it might be something you could look into more if you

have the time.

October 19, Thursday, My response to Adam

Hi Adam, Thanks for the information. I will look her up. Everyone commented on Trenton's t-shirt you got him. They want to take a picture with him in it. Kind of funny.

I think I should do speeches on the importance of having insurance. I tell you, I don't know what would have happened if we hadn't gotten catastrophic for Trenton.

Email from Stephanie

Hi Susan! Can you even believe Trenton will be home in a week??? It really does feel like it's been forever. I bet he's excited and nervous. I'm leaving town next weekend but I think I could make it to the airport. Honestly, do you think he would be ok with that? I'm sure he's gonna be overwhelmed, I'm just guessing, but I think there will be a large crowd! I so can't wait to see him. I hope to come by on that Mon. or Tues. after he gets home cuz I've got something for him and I think Friday will be too crazy, but I would love to be there to welcome him home if you think it's all right. I hope that you are all doing ok. I'm sure at this point you are feeling slightly overwhelmed yourself (understatement). Please let me know what I can do. I'm out on the home improvements but if anything else comes up, I'm here. Looking forward to seeing you all real soon! Take care. Good luck with the travel. Lots of LOVE, Stephanie

October 19, Thursday, Email from Nathan

Hi,

Just wanted to let you know that the concert helped to raise around $1,750. We are waiting on a donation from one other company to hopefully push us to $2,000. Thank you so much for going up on stage and speaking. I know that meant a lot to everyone who was there. You really let everyone know exactly why we were doing this and that was very important to me. I am hoping to make this a yearly event and each year getting bigger and bigger bands. I graduate this year, but I will probably come back to do the event, or at least help with it. Just wanted to let you know what was going on.

My response to Nathan
Hi Nathan,

I just read Trenton your email and he was so appreciative. You all were amazing, especially you. What a great job you did. I can't thank you enough for this. We really had a good time and we were so glad we could be there. If I can ever help in any way, I would love to. Thanks again Nathan; it was so good to finally meet you and again, you are awesome.

Email from Chip and Deanna (friends from BOMA)
Hi Susan,

I've been keeping tabs on Trenton and his progress through various sources, but just recently received your e-mail address. First, I want you to know you have been in our prayers since the accident and we have been wishing for nothing but positive news right from the start. Secondly, I can only imagine how tough this has been on you, as well as Rick and the girls, but especially you. You all have done so well with Trenton and we wish for you the strength to keep everything as positive as possible for all of you.

I read that Trenton is scheduled to return to K.C. next week and that is wonderful news. I'm not at all surprised that he wants to be on his own with his friends, but you are right, he'll need full time help in getting acclimated to his new world.

How did the party on the 22nd go? I bet it was overwhelmingly successful. When you get a chance, let us know how things are going, OK? In the meantime, our best wishes are with you all....

October 24, Tuesday, Email to Jane
Jane,

Please understand that when we are in these monthly conferences I bring up all these concerns and more and I am told by the doctor, PT, OT, social worker and whoever else is in there that it is taken care of. Regardless, I still have been contacting the tech guy and I have told him that the #1 priority is to get him a totally voice-activated phone so he can say "911". I also am not comfortable with him being there at all by himself, but again the "team" says if Trenton wants to try it, to let him.

Again, we do not plan on him being by himself at all initially. I have concerns with the roommate situation and have ordered every tape imaginable and they will watch it so they are aware of any situation that does not look right.

I know you are concerned and love Trenton very much. That is not an issue. We are all stressed but we are trying to think of everything and still know we are not going to make it perfect. I am not opposed to advice, someone to talk to or any help. And when I said I knew all this it did not mean that I was all knowing, just that I, too, am aware and concerned about everything. The last thing I need is to have everyone upset with me.

Part of the reason I am so stressed is knowing how hard this is going to be when Trenton comes home. He thinks he is ready but I am not sure he is emotionally. I leave Thursday and we arrive Friday. I know Trenton wants to see everyone. I don't want to fight but you are right, I am pretty strung out right now, as we all are.

Jane's response
Susan,

I certainly DID NOT mean to upset you Thursday night on the phone. I never have been critical of the way you have handled this dreadful situation. I know these past four months have been your worst nightmare and it is not over yet. I realize that on one hand Trenton coming home is a relief, but on the other it brings a whole new set of concerns and problems. I also do not pretend to have the RIGHT answers to any of this. How could I know when I am not in your shoes and do not know all the specifics about what is needed for Trenton's home care?

All I was trying to do was to "process" information with you. I do think that you are so stretched emotionally that it would only make sense that talking to someone a little removed from all of this could be helpful. I understand to some degree Trenton's care will be trial and error in determining what exactly is needed. That is why I am concerned that Trenton's roommates move in immediately. I was just thinking that if he ends up needing more home nursing care in the beginning, just to get settled in, and if you, Ashley, or Rick end up wanting to spend the night for the first couple of weeks or so, that extra bedroom could be available. The people that Angela has talked to all agree that this is going to be a very difficult time for Trenton. I know he thinks he is anxious to have roommates again, but remember he told you that he feels he has to put up a good front for his friends? He obviously will have a lot of adjusting to do and trying to save face with his friends just might be an additional stressor, even if he does not see that now. I could go on about some other concerns I have based on what Angela has been told but it seems you would rather I not do that.

Susan, I love Trenton and even though my pain is minor compared to yours as his mother, these past four months have been hard on his extended family as well. We all wish we could turn back time. We all pray for a miracle every day and BELIEVE that he will get one.

I know you are under unbelievable stress but please do not make me feel like I am making things worse for you. Do you honestly think I would want to do that? Again, I was only trying to "process" information from a more objective viewpoint. I was not trying to add stress to your life, nor did I need you making me feel like I was doing so.

I plan on being at the airport on Friday. Let me know if there is anything that needs to be done to be ready for Trenton.

My extended family was worried about you living on your own with two roommates. I was worried about it. I know everything said was out of love and good intention. But, I was stuck. You were a 24-year-old young man who had lost nearly all your independence. You didn't want to live with your Mom and I didn't blame you. Was I worried? YES! Could I do anything about it? Sure. I could force the issue and make you live with me and then you would have been more miserable. I couldn't do that to you.

Email from Sam

Susan,

Please thank your son for embarrassing me this week in fantasy football. I thought about calling him today but wasn't sure how busy things are, this being his last week at the hospital.

If you need any help getting Trenton settled/moved in this week please let me know -- I am free most of the week.

My response to Sam

Hey Sam,

I will let him know, but he hasn't done too well himself in fantasy football. We are going to move the furniture tomorrow if Ashley gets off work. If you can help that would be great. If you want to give me yours, I can call you to let you know for sure if it is tomorrow. Won't be too much just some furniture. We got his clothes over last night. Thanks Sam.

October 26, Thursday, Update from Me

Hi there,

Just wanted to reiterate if you would like to see Trenton, we arrive on Friday, the 28th, United Flight #1246 at 12:45pm. He will be the last one off the plane so it may take a while. I know he is anxious to see everyone. Thanks and see you soon.

Email from Ryan

I am sure Trenton told you but I was out there this weekend and I had such a good time with Trenton...he is doing so well and everyone I have talked to is so excited to have Trenton back in KC. I was talking to Ashley on Friday and she mentioned some type of website about Missouri and Stem Cell Research...I was wondering if you had that website. Thanks so much and I am sure I will see you around more now that Trenton will be back home.

My response to Ryan

Hi Ryan,

Yes, Trenton was so glad to see you.

The website is <u>www.MissouriCures.com.</u> We are excited to get him home and a little nervous, as I know he is. Feel free to come over whenever you'd like.

Trenton is back in Kansas City after four months!

October 30, Monday, Update from Me

Hi all,

First of all, thanks to so many of you who welcomed Trenton back on Friday. He is thrilled to be back. The Thursday night before leaving Craig, we went out to ESPN Zone with Courtney, Brandi and a few of his other favorites. John, who lives in Colorado and who has been wonderful about visiting the times he knew no one was with him, also joined us. It was emotional saying goodbye, especially to Courtney, but they have promised to do a road trip and come to see us maybe the first weekend in December. We were up at 5:00 am on Friday getting ready for the plane ride home. The checking in and security went fairly smoothly. The only snag was Rick lost his Blackberry when doing a weight shift with Trenton. We also did not transfer him from his manual chair to the aisle wheelchair like we were supposed to, but we got him on and off the plane, which is what counted. Trenton fell asleep immediately and slept the entire flight home.

We got him settled in the house and he loves it. His friends have been amazing, as we knew they would be, and have been this entire time. We still have quite a few things to get worked out and hopefully some sort of a routine will fall into place.

Rick, Ashley, Tyson, Jamie, myself, and especially Trenton, want to thank you all again for your friendship and support during this time. One of the aides since we have been back told me she thought Trenton's injury happened a year ago in June because she thought he was doing so well for only four months since the injury. We all believe Trenton will continue to improve each day, and with his amazing attitude, achieve his goals.

I am thinking this might be a good stopping point for the updates but I appreciate you all for allowing me to share his progress with you. Please feel free anytime to email me if you want some news. As

I have said, we are blessed with so many great friends.

Thanks so much again for everything. We know we still have a very long road ahead of us but it helps to know we can count on our friends.

Email from Susie

Susan,

I just wanted to tell you how great it was to see Trenton Friday and the progress he has made. He obviously has been working very hard! I know you have too, right along with him!

I was just wondering how things are going? Is the house going to work out okay and did you get to take Trenton to that horrible football game yesterday?

Please know that I will continue to keep Trenton, you and your family in my prayers!

My email to Susie

Hi Susie,

Thanks, it is good to have him home and he was so excited to see everyone. I will have to take a picture of him with Allison's blanket on. He has it on constantly and loves it. Things are actually going pretty well. When we first got to his place, the Visiting Nurse Assn. called and said that they did not do the things we needed (don't ask me why, have no idea) so I had to go to a private agency that Angela had looked into and now we have CNAs coming in around the clock until we can figure out how much we need. It is hard on Trenton not having a good routine yet, but it will take some time. I filled his prescriptions yesterday and for a month it was $700.00. I could not believe it. His house is going to work out well and I am thrilled with Sam and Chris. They tell everyone to leave when it gets late etc. and are willing to help, which is wonderful. We are getting ready to go over for the games. Thanks so much for everything. Let's go out sometime. Maybe we can get Nancy, Vicki and have some fun. Speaking of fun, they did go to the game yesterday. I didn't, as he needed too many things, so I just ran errands. Talk to you soon.

Allison's email to me

Hi Susan,

Thanks for the email, I would still love to get updates on Trenton's adjustment to KC and progress! It was soooo good to see Trenton on Friday! He looked so good. How did he do going to the NWMSU game on Saturday? I was thinking about him. Is he excited to be back, or a little nervous? Does he have his dog at the house, or not because I was thinking sometime that I could stop by and bring my puppy, Cooper, to play with his dog? I really want to come by his house and see him. What is the best way to get in touch with someone to make sure it's okay to come over? I'm at work, so I probably better actually get back to working, but just wanted to drop a line. Just let me know how to get ahold of someone to come over because I was thinking about early next week sometime! Talk soon, let me know if you need anything.

My email to Allison

Hi Allison,

Trenton loves his Believe blanket. He is so funny because he gets so cold and is wearing the blanket a lot. Thanks so much. And for someone who doesn't sew, you did an awesome job! When you do go over to visit, be prepared and wear summer wear.

Someone will be at his house all the time so anytime would work. He usually gets up around 9:00, so any time after that. He does not have Willy all the time yet and I'm not sure how that will go. Willy was glad to see him though. Please bring Cooper. I'm sure Trenton would love to see him.

He did go to the game and I think they had a good time. I ended up not going, just ran errands all day.

Any one of us should be there, plus an aide is usually there until we get things figured out.

Thanks for being so wonderful. Please stop by anytime.

Email from Vicki (friend of mine)

Morning Susan, just wanted to say what a wonderful job you did of sending out the updates. I'm sure there were many times when that was the last thing you felt like doing, but they are always the first thing I read every day when I open my e-mail and it was great to be able to stay up-to-date on what was happening with Trenton. So, thanks very much.

Philip and Jess watched part of the Chiefs game at Trenton's yesterday and Philip said the house was AWESOME. He's off work today and he's planning on going over to watch a movie with Trenton later on.

As always, if there's anything we can do, don't hesitate to ask.

My response to Vicki
Hi Vicki,

I am so excited for you. Congratulations on the engagement. I saw Philip and his girlfriend over at Trenton's. They are so cute. Anyway, I love planning fun stuff so if you need any help, call me. We are trying to get settled. Just a few glitches, but for the most part, not bad. Very good to get him home.

How is everything with you? How is work? I am working but my mind is not back into it yet; just constantly worried.

Email from Babs (friend of mine)
Dear Susan,

Thank you for all of Trenton's updates. He and you all have been in my prayers since the accident and will continue to be. I wore a blue "Trenton" bracelet daily. When the girl who does my nails asked about it, she was so touched by his story that she went and bought one too and has not taken it off. I know the journey continues and my prayers are for everyone's strength, patience, and courage to continue.

My response to Babs
Hi Babs,

Thanks so much for the thoughts and prayers and I loved hearing about the bracelet. We have been so fortunate to have such great people around us. We are still trying to get some things worked out with the care he is getting but I'm sure it will just take some time. Thanks again and I hope all is well with you.

Email from Angela (high school friend of yours)
Susan,

I am so glad that the trip home was so good for you all. Tell Trenton I am sorry I could not come to the airport to greet him home. Unfortunately, I could not get off work. Hopefully you guys are getting settled back in K.C. Well, I would really like to come and visit Trenton. Let me know when is good for you guys. Hope to see you all soon.

My response
Hi Angela,

Please feel free to visit Trenton any time. The neighborhood is Grey Oaks right behind Oak Park High School soccer fields. Thanks and keep in touch.

Email from Libby

I don't want the updates to end, even though I know it takes a lot of time and energy from you! I don't get a chance to talk to you that often, and like hearing about his progress.

David isn't set on where he is going to school - touring MU was just a starting point. So we will see....let me know how things progress, or if I can do anything for you all or Trenton. Don't know what it would be, unless maybe cooking. Let me know if you get tired of cooking for the guys!

My response to Libby

It really does not take that much time and I enjoyed doing them but I don't want to wear people out with my updates. We are having a bit of trouble with the home health but it will work out.

I imagine David could go just about anywhere he wanted to so I'm sure he has lots to think about.

Email from Lindsay
Hey Susan,

Wow - I know this past week has been super busy for you, but it sounds like everything is coming together. You should be proud. You all have taken Trenton a long way since June. I can't wait to get home and see his new place. Do you have his new address by chance? My aunt Linda wanted to send Trenton something for his new place, and I could use it as well.

Caleb and his buddy, Danny, have been talking to Rick the past couple days, getting the whole Chiefs thing worked out. From what I gather, they are going to get him to a private Friday practice where he can actually mingle with the players without them being distracted by the upcoming game. It should all work out great.

My response to Lindsay

Hi Lindsay,

The Chiefs thing sounds wonderful. I know Trenton will have a great time. He seems to be doing well. It was emotional leaving Craig and emotional coming home, so basically I am emotional all the time, as I am sure you have heard. I'm sure I will even out eventually. Hopefully, I won't have alienated all my friends and family in the meantime. Take care and I will see you soon. Can't believe Thanksgiving is so close.

Email from Adam

Things have been hectic at work lately. I really miss college, lol. Growing up has its pros and cons. Take your time on the tape, I know you are super busy and things have to be very hectic with all the new stuff going on in Trenton's life. How is Jamie doing in Columbia? Is she holding up well? If you can also give me Trenton's cell phone if he has it yet or give Trenton my cell phone. I have really enjoyed calling him up and chatting with him. I try and call every 4 to 5 days or so. Just want to keep in touch. I talked to him about going skydiving, because our reservation for it fell through. I still have a voucher though. I think he says he has a voucher also. He said he is going to look into it. Hope all is well and hope Trenton is getting used to being home. Did he go to the game and have fun? He told me he was going when I talked to him on Wednesday. Anyways, got to go. Talk to you soon.

My response to Adam

I just got word that Trenton's phone will be hooked up as of

Friday, 6:00 p.m. This is not his voice activated phone, at least not yet, but at least it is a land line. I am meeting with a tech guy and hopefully getting him voice-activated.

I don't know. The thought of him jumping from an airplane right now does not excite me too much. He really can't break anything else. Would not be good.

Jamie likes MU pretty well. Can't get below a C on any tests but I told her the 1st semester they try to weed out kids and be happy with that for right now. I think it is good for her to be away from some of this and just have some fun.

I think it is hard when you first get out of college. All of a sudden you are expected to be responsible and get a job, and where did all the fun go? Take care and I will get you the picture of Trenton wearing the t-shirt you got him.

So, let me explain the reference from the above email from Adam regarding skydiving. You had gotten this as a Christmas present from your dad prior to the accident. After your accident your dad had called to see if you would still be able to go. The thought of your skydiving right now was not very appealing to me. I told your dad that I did not want you up in an airplane and then jumping out of it anytime soon.

Email from Jane

I cannot open my e-card but I understand it is pretty funny. I am forwarding it to school so hopefully it will open there tomorrow.

I know this past weekend was stressful. Trenton seems to be getting along great and that is the main thing. Ashley seems to be getting things squared away with the home health care people.

As I tried to say in my last email to you, I do not pretend to know what is best for Trenton. I do think, because I am not as emotionally drained as you are, I can see things from a different perspective. Talking things through with others always helps me when making tough decisions. That is all I was trying to do Thursday night.

Trenton's accident and his condition has been difficult for ALL members of this family. We all want what is best for him and want to help anyway we can. Please accept our thoughts, questions, and suggestions as acts of concern, not criticism. We love you and only want to do what we can to make things easier.

Email from Mary Alice

Dear Susan,

God is just good, isn't He? Please don't remove me from the list. I think of all of you so often, and love knowing how things are progressing.

I think you all have just done remarkably well, considering all the things you've had to cope with. Obviously, you have a good circle of friends who love and take care of you.

I hope you're able to rest a bit now - sometimes the aftermath is almost harder to deal with. When you're so busy, it doesn't give you time to dwell on things as much as when life has slowed down a bit.

We're looking forward to having the girls (and son-in-law) home for Thanksgiving. Jenny is totally stressed, on overload, senior-itis - papers due, etc. Melissa has just been accepted into a Master's program in English, so we're excited about that. More excited that we don't have to pay for this one.

Email from Kathy (mother from Springfield, MO whose son had lost his arm and leg)

Hi Susan,

I just wanted to check and see how Trenton is getting along at home. We have all been thinking of him and wishing him well. Just as we have experienced with Barry, it takes a lot of adjustment at first. I know you must worry a lot with him living on his own, but I have learned with Barry that a little independence goes a long way for attitude and mood improvement. I was a nervous wreck the first few times he left the house with his friends, and especially when he started driving again. Everyone finally convinced me that he needed to build his confidence, but it's still hard not to worry.

Barry is still walking, driving, and even working a few hours a week with his prosthetic leg. In the last few weeks, however, it's been giving him some trouble. An X-ray with the orthopedic surgeon confirmed that he has developed a bone spur on the end of his leg which is causing the pain when he walks with his prosthesis. So, we are scheduled for same-day surgery next Tuesday to have the spur removed. They said it won't take long, we can come home the same day, and he should be able to start wearing his leg again in about two weeks. It sure messed up our Thanksgiving plans, but we have to look at the big picture and get him back to walking without pain ASAP.

Other than that, he's doing great. He already has much more use of his shoulder and arm than they originally thought, and it continues to improve. They are thinking that he will have a much better chance of a functional prosthetic arm than they originally thought. In the meantime, physical therapy is working wonders for it.

My response to Kathy
Hi Kathy,

I was just saying I needed to write you. We did get Trenton home. It was very emotional leaving Craig. It was a security issue. As much as I wanted him home I was a nervous wreck because I knew his care was in our hands now. He is in his own little villa type house with two roommates. Home health has been a nightmare but we have one that is pretty good and I am still interviewing and looking for others. It is amazing what agencies send to you. He has care from 11pm to 11am and then one of his roommates does not have a job right now and he has been wonderful. Helps us out a lot. Hopefully, by the time he gets a job, we will have Trenton's voice activation phone etc. in place and he can be alone for about five hours during the day. As you know, they so want to be independent as much as possible. I can't imagine having someone with me all the time. His spirits are still amazing and his outlook is fairly positive. I think he has done better than any of us.

I am so glad to hear Barry is doing so well. Can you believe we have been living this for five months? Don't you wonder how you ever got through it and how you still are? I hope all goes well with the surgery. It is always something, isn't it? I think that is the hardest part, knowing there is always an issue, a health concern etc. Mentally it is very hard to get a break.

I do have good news. My oldest daughter, Ashley, just found out she is pregnant and we are thrilled. She has already looked into blood cord freezing for Trenton down the road. You never lose hope, which is a good thing.

It is always good to hear from you. Try to have a good holiday and lots of luck next Tuesday.

Email from Ryan

I am not sure if Trenton will be getting home health from physical therapy but if he ever needs to be stretched, I would be more than happy to help out. If a therapist does come to his home every week, I am sure that will be sufficient but if not, let me know and we can try to set up a schedule. Talk to you later.

My response to Ryan

Hi Ryan,

Good to hear from you. Right now we are having such a time getting good nursing care, as I'm sure you can imagine. Honestly, I don't know where some of these people come from. Trenton is hanging in there but a little frustrated. I would love for you to work with him some and I know he would too. If you have time, anytime would be great. Just let me know.

Email from Adam

Hey Susan,

Thanks a lot for sending me that picture. I really like it. He looks really happy. How is he adjusting to his new home? Is he getting along well? Does he have a cell phone yet I can call, or his only phone the house phone at this house?

Hope all is well, I will be home during Thanksgiving. Do you think Trenton will have time to visit? I would love to see his place. Don't know if you guys are going to be busy with family stuff that weekend. I will be home for like four or five days. Are you guys staying in town for that? If he has a cell number shoot it my way when you have time. Thanks again for the picture, it is awesome. I have it in a frame in my office. Seems like he had some really cool nurses.

My response to Adam

Hi Adam,

I am glad you liked the picture. Trenton loves his house but finding good nursing care is a nightmare and very frustrating. Hopefully it will work out. His phone is not working yet and does not have the voice activated one either. Hopefully this week we will get something worked out and I will send out his phone # then.

We will be home Thanksgiving and Trenton would love to see you. Anytime. He lives right behind the Oak Park soccer field in an addition called Grey Oaks. You have my #, just call, but he is almost always there. Looking forward to seeing you. Have a good week.

Email from Carolyn (friend of mine)

Hi Susan,

I just wanted to say thanks for all your good communications about Trenton. It was so nice to be able to keep up to date.

Good luck to all of you now that Trenton is home. It will be so much easier on all of you to have him close. What is his new address, by the way? I hope you settle into a good routine and that Trenton keeps improving. I thought he looked great, and it sounds like the professionals are pretty impressed with his progress too. It was so good to see him and welcome him home, even though he probably thought "who in the heck are those strangers?"

My response to Carolyn

Hi Carolyn,

Thank you for all your support. We very much appreciate it. We are still adjusting and I imagine we will be for a while. Nursing care is a nightmare but hopefully we will get it taken care of soon. Poor Trenton, he is pretty patient but very frustrated.

Thanks again and let's keep in touch. I will send out occasional emails as he progresses.

Email from Barbara (friend of mine)

Hi Susan

Just wanted to let you know how much I enjoyed your updates on Trenton and how I miss them. I'm sure you're ready to move on but I just wanted to let you know how much I looked forward to hearing from you. So many times people just send jokes and cartoons but your taking the time every day to put your thoughts down was generous.

I know it's not your job to educate the rest of us, but I just wondered if you would consider writing once in a while to let us know how things are going. I'm sure you're thinking, "Yeah, I've got time for that @#$!" Anyhow, hope you and Trenton got to go to the Chief's game yesterday. What a game! For once, it was even on TV in Saint Louis since the Rams weren't playing this week.

Anyhow, just wanted to drop you a line and let you know how much your emails meant and that we're thinking about you and yours. If there is anything we can do, please don't hesitate to ask. So far, my work schedule is pretty light for the rest of the month and so far for December.

My response to Barb
Hi Barb,

Thanks and I appreciate that very much. I will write updates every once in a while. I just didn't want to bore anyone with his day to day activities. Right now we have had nursing care nightmares but hopefully we will get it worked out. Trenton didn't go to the game yesterday. He gets so cold; it is just easier for him to watch it at home. His spirits are pretty good; just frustrated with the nursing care.

How are you all doing? I miss seeing the old tailgate group. I went over for a while yesterday. What a good game!

Back in Kansas City on October 28, 2005

So, we got you home on a Friday and on Saturday night Terresa and Mike were getting married. You really wanted to go. I was invited to the wedding as well, so Ric 2 and I were going to take you. When we arrived to your house you were ready; however, I noticed your pants were wet as well as the wheelchair seat cushion. Apparently your catheter bag had become kinked, causing it to leak. You told me not to worry about it and that you just wouldn't go to the wedding. There was no way that was going to happen so I got you in the Hoyer lift and out of your chair and into the bed. I then proceeded to climb all over you to get you out of the wet pants and into dry clothes using strategically placed towels. I took the seat cover off the cushion of the wheelchair and rinsed it out, dried it and put the cushion back into the chair. Now to get you into the chair.

I got you back in the Hoyer lift and lowered you to just above the cushion and then set you in the chair. I remove the sling and you slide right off the chair. I grab you and put you right back on and you slide right off again. I am thinking WTF; what is wrong with this thing? Ric 2 is trying to help me, but he knows less about it than I do, but at this point he is at least keeping you from falling to the ground while I am checking out what could be wrong. Finally, I realize that the cushion was turned around. So I get it on correctly and put you back in the seat, where you thankfully stay. You are good, but my hair is plastered to my face and my clothes feel like they are part of my skin from sweating, even though it is the end of October. No matter. We load up in the car and off we go.

We are at the reception and all your friends are talking to you and so glad to see you. I am truly happy, as this is the first time you have seen some of your friends since the accident. I see Rick and Cathy and they look wonderful. And I lost it. I wasn't mad at

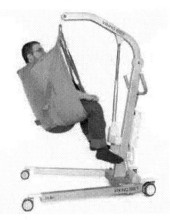

them, but I was frustrated. They had no idea what it took to get you there that night. Of course, I went off where no one could see me, but I was tired and knew I looked a mess and just lost it. I had already sweated off most of my makeup so a few tears didn't really change the way I looked. Thankfully, I recovered and no one had a clue.

A Hoyer lift.

It was wonderful getting you home and it also scared me to death. Chris and Sam were going to be living with you to help with meals etc., but we needed nursing care. We were also told by the staff at Craig it was important to keep you stretched. It was also my understanding you would need to be turned fairly frequently during the night to help prevent skin breakdown. I wondered how all of this was going to be possible when you refused to live with family. And, as mentioned, my family was also wondering the same thing and was pretty vocal about it. At that time you had medications that had to be given in the morning, noon, 5 p.m. and evening. While I knew everyone was trying to be helpful, it was also extremely stressful. I was getting advice (unsolicited) from everyone. No one believed I knew what I was doing and they were right.

Again, Children's Mercy, aka Silvia, was wonderful. She allowed me the time off I needed to do what you would let me do. I had found someone who would do aquatic therapy at the North Kansas City Hospital Rehabilitation Pool. You didn't especially like it because when you were done I would have to get you dressed for the day and back into your chair. I tried to be very respectful of your privacy and felt I did a pretty good job with it. While you were very thin at that time, you are still a tall man and it was difficult for me to lift you to get dressed. I literally would be contorted in the craziest positions and honestly exhausted by the time I got you back in your chair. You were also cold after the water therapy and it took you awhile to warm up. You hung in there for several months and then you were done with the aquatic therapy.

Cold was a big problem for you at that time. You would have us put a blanket over your head and then turn on your space heater and then tell us you were good and we could go now. I tried to comply, but honestly it scared me to death leaving you with a blanket over your head and a space heater on. I also felt at this point you didn't care what happened to you. I'd get you settled and then try to not think about you as I went through the rest of the day. Of course, this was impossible. I thought about you every waking minute. Worry, fear, and tears were part of my daily activities. I didn't know how to be okay again. Ashley and Jamie wanted their mother back, Ric 2 wanted his girlfriend back, my sisters and friends wanted their sister/ friend back. While my work was very understanding, I needed to work.

Friends and family were still very eager to help out. So, another one of my brainy (and I am sure annoying) ideas was to have a schedule for stretching and meals. I am not sure if I discussed this with you first, but I was truly thinking I was doing the right thing. So, for a while (and again I think it was pretty short- lived), people were coming and going and cooking and feeding and stretching. I completely understand now that this had to have been so difficult for you. Some of these people you really didn't know that well. I know there were days you didn't feel like seeing anyone, much less having them feed you and stretch you and make idle conversation. Plus, we didn't truly know what we were doing, so sometimes the stretching hurt and you were honestly too kind to say much. While you were amazed and truly appreciative of the support of everyone, having people coming and going all day long was uncomfortable for you. I think about this now and I truly feel horrible I had not been more sensitive at the time of your feelings and privacy.

Getting help for your showers and bathroom needs was a

nightmare. We tried agencies first. Of course these people get paid next to nothing, so unfortunately they are uneducated and most have had a very rough life. We were told by the agency their employees were very well trained to work with quadriplegics. Of course, they were not. And most of the ones they sent over you didn't want to train. I honestly can't remember how many we went through before we had two trained and with you for some time.

Why Kennedy Krieger Institute in Baltimore?

When you were first injured, Lindsay, your cousin, had learned about Dr. John McDonald, a neurologist, in Baltimore, Maryland. Dr. McDonald is the director of the International Center for Spinal Cord Injury at Kennedy Krieger. He had launched a spinal cord rehabilitation and research program. You were interested in going, so we began the process of getting you there.

At this time, you had two caregivers who were fairly dependable and trustworthy. They did work for an agency, but they would tell their employer they were going to take vacation during your time at Kennedy Krieger. While your dad and I could stay with you in Baltimore, we still needed your caregivers with us to provide your personal needs. I am sure the agency knew, but they never said anything.

We would be with these girls for one to two weeks at a time. Trina came with us most of the time. She was a sweet girl in her 20s. She had a son and they lived with her father. Trina's look was very suggestive. She wore her shirts very tight with her breasts exposed. She was a tiny girl, though she consumed a lot of food. I did her laundry in Baltimore and I could barely fit my arm in her pant leg. Her makeup was heavy--bright blue eyeshadow and a lot of it. Without makeup she was actually quite pretty and childlike.

I never knew exactly what had happened with Trina in her childhood, though she did talk about her mother some, and not favorably. She said she had been a cutter. At the time, I didn't know what that meant and had to look it up.

So, everyone noticed Trina. She also had an oral fixation and was constantly chewing on coffee straws or she would sit and eat mustard or sugar packets. I had never seen anything like it. During these trips I am sure we looked pretty funny. I knew you were mortified and it was during this time that you let your beard grow really long and you wore a hat. When waiting for the flight you would ask me to pull your hat down and the blanket up over your face. Of course, doing anything with a quadriplegic draws attention, which was the last thing you wanted.

Getting on a plane is arduous and involves a lot of help. You would board first. Southwest Airlines was/is wonderful in every aspect of your travel. You would get yourself down the jetway in your power chair and then the Southwest Airlines staff would put you in an aisle chair. This aisle chair is literally as wide as the aisle so not wide! They strap you in and get you on the plane. Then they have to lift you into a chair. I then have a strap that I put around your chest and through the chair's food tray behind you so you would be able to stay upright. You would then be the last person to get off the plane.

Once we would get to Baltimore I would have ordered a van to get you to the Residence Inn where we were staying. Now we tried many things during your trips to Baltimore. Once your Dad drove you out in your van with all of your equipment. This was nice because you didn't have to get up at the crack of dawn to catch the van to Kennedy Krieger every day and we didn't have to search high and low for a Hoyer lift, shower chair and any other equipment you might need. Also, loading a 500 lb. power wheel chair in an airplane is not great on a chair. However, the drive was difficult, to say the least. Your Dad ran into all kinds of weather and it really wasn't great on you to be in your chair for such a long time.

We would stay at a Residence Inn in Baltimore and they were wonderful. The best scenario for me was a two bedroom with a living room in between. We had a small one bedroom one time that was honestly awful. I don't think I slept the entire time I was there. I gave Trina the sofa and I slept on the floor. There was nowhere to go to "get away" for a while.

The staff at Kennedy Krieger was exceptional. I was convinced every physical and occupational therapist in the world was smart, kind and cute. They would work with you all day. Sometimes they would have outings and we would get together with them later. I was sold on the therapy, but not so much on Baltimore. I had been to

Baltimore before, but I had never driven there. I think I mentioned earlier I am the worst with directions and often I would get turned around. Very calmly you would say to me, "Mom, see those blue lights on the streets?" And I would acknowledge those lights and you would tell me this meant we were in the worst part of Baltimore and to get our asses out of there.

The first time we travelled to Baltimore with Trina I did wonder a bit about her eating habits. I may have said to you I didn't understand how she remained so skinny when she ate so much. You didn't want to talk about Trina so you didn't say anything. On our second trip it finally dawned on me what was going on. Our room had a kitchenette so we would get some food to have on hand for breakfast and snacking. The Residence Inn also had a full breakfast and dinner every day. I think dinner went from 5-7pm. We would get back from therapy and you would rest for a while. Around 5:30 or so you would be ready for dinner so I would go down, fix you a plate and bring it up. Trina would head down around 6 and be down there until dinner shut down. She would eat the entire time she was down there and then would come back up with plate loads of French fries, pasta, meat; you name, it she had it. Staff took a liking to her and would let her take all the leftover food back to our room and she would proceed to eat it all. I kid you not. All of it. She would then get in the refrigerator freezer and pull out a frozen pizza and cook it. Around 8ish she would head to the shower and an hour later she would emerge. If she was awake she was either eating or had something in her mouth.

I had never seen anything like it. How on earth could this skinny, tiny person eat all this food? I remember texting pretty much everyone I knew one night and said, "Eating every fucking thing in sight." I failed to put Trina and not me so everyone thought I was having a meltdown. I clarified that no, it was not me, but Trina. I was so naïve at first, as I had no idea she was bulimic. Once I realized, I was horrified as to what she must be doing to her body. I did try to talk to her and I truly wanted to help her. But, honestly, I was a little overwhelmed as it was. She seemed close to her father and she was crazy about her son. One morning we were sitting in occupational therapy waiting for the therapists to get started and

Trina was on the floor with two straws hanging from her mouth. She looked like a walrus. This was after she had put 10 sugar packs in her coffee.

The caregivers had never been on a plane or in another city. Because we were so close to DC and it was easy to get to by train, I asked Trina if she wanted to go to DC. I knew they had a sightseeing tour you could catch right from the train station. She was very excited and had a great day. A few years later Trina passed away. She hadn't been working for you for a couple of years. It was, and is, still very sad to me.

We also had CiCi. CiCi was scary. Just plain rough. She cussed like a sailor and she would just as soon tell you to go fuck yourself. I didn't even try to talk about her past. Truly, she scared me. I also offered for her to go to DC and she was very excited to do this as well. I did encourage CiCi to be polite to anyone she came into contact with and discouraged her from cussing anyone out. I told her she could get into a lot of trouble and she needed to be nice. She didn't work for you too much longer after that and I have no idea what ever became of her.

Baltimore was good for you. You met a lot of nice people. You haven't been for several years and much of the reason has been because of your health. I know you would like to go back and I would love to see you go back.

Maneuvering Tight Spaces

As you had pointed out to us in Springfield, you had lost a tooth in the accident. You wanted it replaced with a permanent tooth so once you got home we began the process. This is a fairly lengthy process and required a few trips to the dentist. It was during one of those trips that I pulled up in front of the building and put down the ramp to get you out. For some reason (and that reason escapes me now) you weren't using your sip and puff to get out of the van. I was trying to hold this 500 lb. chair, because if I let it go, I could tell your fingers were going to hit the door and bend all the way back. Of course, I couldn't hold that chair and I remember yelling, "Sorry" and let go. You were fine, but I was a mess. I then parked the car and you are now using the sip and puff heading to the door of the building. Your wheel gets caught in the rocks and you can't get out on your own. It is quite obvious at this point I am unable to do much with that 500 lb. chair, so a Good Samaritan came along and helped you out. You then proceeded to the door. Unfortunately, the door frame is not quite wide enough, and you end up dislodging the door frame, but you are able to catch a fairly tall floor plant, so in you go with the frame ajar and the plant following you. Oh my God, I am half hysterical laughing and crying at this point. The dentist sees us and was amazing. Without skipping a beat she looks at the door and says, "We were going to replace that door anyway."

You were also struggling with ingrown toenails during this time. So again, we would go to these appointments and maneuver your way into these very tight buildings. It truly at times was like a bull in a china shop. Once your feet got better and you could wear somewhat normal shoes, you had Sam take you to Dick's Sporting Goods to get you tennis shoes. You were tooling around in your chair when a sales guy (young) came up to you and asked if he could help you. You looked at him with a very serious face and requested, "Your best pair of running shoes." I guess the look on his face was priceless.

You have always had a great sense of humor and have always been self-deprecating. You are not one that typically likes a lot of attention. Now you can't go anywhere without drawing attention. People do stare, and while I get frustrated with it sometimes, you are so kind to everyone around you. For a while you did some public speaking. You would go to schools and talk about your accident. After one of your talks to a classroom of young people, maybe age 6 or 7, the teacher had them write thank yous to you for speaking. Most drew pictures with their note. The cutest one and the one that made it on your refrigerator was a little boy who drew a picture of a pool and then a stick person splat on the pool bottom. We were pretty sure he understood what you had been trying to tell them.

Your driver's license had expired and in order for you to travel to Baltimore you needed a current ID. We headed to the driver's license bureau and in we go. When it is our turn we go up to the girl who was about the most expressionless girl I have ever encountered. She took your information, had you wheel up to the eye terminal with the traffic signs, etc. Yeah, you passed, so then she has you line up for your picture. She then says in her monotone voice to sign for the new license. OMG; we just look at each other. I look at her and kind of cock my head to one side as if to say, "Really" and "Are you kidding me right now." I mean, seriously, had she even looked at you? She says, "Well, he has to sign it." So, you tell me to put the pen in your mouth, which I do, and there you have your signature. We get back into the van and you look at me and say, "Did I just get a license to drive?" I said, "Yes, you did." Lord, pretty scary, isn't it?

I had gotten this hare brain idea to build a facility that could mirror Kennedy Krieger and you could get therapy right here in Kansas City. My friends were on board and so our mission began. In that mission I realized this is no easy task. Karen and I went to visit a facility called Quest to Walk, which is now Project Walk, in Kansas. I walked in and met the nicest and nicest looking people. So my theory was still intact regarding physical and occupational therapists. This is where I met Chris. After talking to him, the owner Tom and the other therapists, I took you out there to meet them and see the facility. You seemed excited and you started going three times a week. There is no doubt this was beneficial for you. You were making progress and with this and then with periodic visits to Baltimore. You were doing well and you were fairly healthy. Chris is now your brother-in-law and father of your nephew. He is very devoted to what is now called Project Walk and helping those with SCIs.

Paralysis, to those who don't live it, and at least for me before I started living with it, was a picture of Christopher Reeve. A lot of people don't know the difference between a quadriplegic and a paraplegic. Quadriplegia is caused by damage to the brain or the spinal cord at a high level, C1 - C7. The injury causes victims to lose partial or total function of all four limbs. All quadriplegics have, or have had, some kind of finger dysfunction. So, it is not uncommon to have a quadriplegic with fully functional arms, only having their fingers not working. Most spinal cord injuries result in loss of sensation and function below the level of injury, including loss of controlled function of the bladder and bowel.

Your injury is a C4-C5 complete. What this means is that your spinal cord was totally injured. I do not dwell on this, and neither should you or anyone else with a spinal cord injury. The fact is that every day they are making advancements and I refuse to believe that one day you won't be walking.

That being said, there needs to be more awareness of this injury and the consequences of it. I have no idea how to make this happen, but maybe hearing your story will help. I initially thought I would write your memoir because I was pretty sure you didn't remember a lot of this. And, honestly, maybe that is the way you wanted to keep it. It isn't necessarily fun to read about what you went through. But, then I thought about Project Walk and other spinal cord recovery facilities. There aren't that many. It is so expensive to have you go to Baltimore for therapy. Because this injury doesn't affect as many people, there isn't much awareness. It is much more difficult to get national support for 250,000 plus SCIs.

While there aren't as many affected by an SCI, let me tell
you, for those that are, the facts are pretty clear. It is devastating
to the individuals and to those around them, financially and
emotionally. The number one cause of this injury is vehicular
accident, followed by falls, trauma (presumably gunshot wounds and
accidents). A small percentage has an injury like yours, less than
20%. Per one million people, there are approximately 40 cases of
a spinal cord injury. Therein lies the problem with awareness and
funding.

And, you are one of the lucky ones. You have a lot of family
and friends to help and support you. Financially your dad has been
able to provide for you. But, during our trips in Baltimore I met
many families who had little to no support emotionally or financially.
The last few years have not been great for you. You have had a lot
of health problems. In the ten years since your injury I would say
you have had a urinary tract infection (UTI) 99% of the time. You
struggle constantly with kidney stones. This is a side effect of
having a supra pubic catheter. Ironically, you can feel nothing, but
you can tell when you have a UTI. You actually get very ill with
them and have been hospitalized numerous times. It is difficult to
find a doctor that specializes in your injury. You have constant
neck and shoulder pain. As I mentioned earlier, quads cannot cough
normally and it is very difficult for you to vomit. You struggle with
regulating you temperature, swelling, and infections.

You get a new wheelchair every five years. So you have had
two. You just got a new one. Due to your health concerns these last
four years, you have gained a lot of weight. So your chair you have
had for those last five years really didn't fit you the last four. This
only exacerbated your health concerns. It doesn't matter how beat
up your chair is or how much you have outgrown it, you don't get a
new one until it has been five years.

Before getting your most recent chair, the handrests were ripped
in half on your old one. The seat cushion broke down, which caused
a huge pressure ulcer. Your chair was held together sort of by duct
tape. Then your van was on its last leg. None of the handicap
accessible devices worked on the van. We had to manually pull
down the ramp and then we had a brick stashed in the van we would

put under the ramp so it didn't break with the weight of the chair and you in it. The seat locks quit working a long time ago, so we manually locked you down. You have broken nearly every one of your toes getting into the van and turning your chair to get you locked down. Your feet hit the back of the chair. Of course, you can't feel it but your toes are always swollen.

I don't mean to complain. These are just some of the things quads deal with. We were lucky your dad was able to financially afford a van. They are very expensive, especially with the handicap conversion package. Your father recently got you a new (used) one. The other one simply was not safe anymore and no one was comfortable driving it.

It is estimated the average cost for the first year of injury for a quadriplegic is a little over a million dollars and then approximately $200,000 each year after. One of the things I know you worry about is the money. Enough said about money. It is a blessing you are with us and you are worth it.

Pressure Ulcers

Pressure ulcers are biggies. Skin breakdown is sneaky and very difficult to heal. When you first notice a pink spot, the ulcer has already started from the inside. Your ulcer on your buttocks was very severe. You had surgery twice for debridement, the medical removal of dead, damaged orinfected tissue to improve healing. However, what we didn't know initially and found out later, was a sponge had been left in the wound, making recovery that much longer and arduous. We don't know who left the sponge in and we never will know. But because of the ulcer you have been in bed for nearly four years.

Some of that time was spent at Kindred, a post acute care facility. You have been there several times off and on and it is not your favorite place. The last time you were there you spent six weeks. While in Kindred, you liked family to come with dinner. It was difficult for you, and understandably so, to have strangers feeding you. We actually talked about this once and you said you were uncomfortable asking them to wash their hands before feeding you. I told you this is a valid request and that no one should have a problem with it. Still I understood your feelings on this. So, on the days I would bring you dinner, and as soon as you were done eating, you would ask me to get the nurse because it was time for your pain medication. You would then tell me I could go home. Not only would you tell me to go home, but you would tell me I do way too much and I needed to take time out for myself. You made me promise to go home and shut everything off and just relax from 7 pm on. While it was nice to think you were really concerned about my well-being, I knew you were hooked on the pain meds and wanted me out of there. There was nothing I could do about it at the time. I knew you would have to deal with it sooner or later so I didn't say anything.

A few days after you came home from Kindred, Nancy informed me she had been up with you all night because you had decided to quit the pain meds cold turkey. Not only was this dangerous, it was also not necessary. I got my stuff and came over and you didn't try to stop me. During the day it wasn't quite as bad, but at night it was just plain awful. You couldn't get comfortable, and for someone that can't move, there isn't much anyone can do. I would adjust the pillows, fans, put cold washcloths on your face, adjust the pillows again, and take the washcloths off your face. When I got you settled and thought you could maybe sleep for a while I went to the sofa just outside of your bedroom. About every ten minutes you yelled out, "Mom," "Fuck," and this went on through the night. I would get into the room and you'd asked me if you had yelled for me. I said you were repeatedly saying, "Fuck" and "Mom" and I didn't know if they were meant to mean the same thing, but I came in regardless. It wasn't like I could do much when I did come in. Sometimes you had me put the towel back on your forehead and sometimes I just sat with you for a while. It took you several days to feel better. I knew the pain meds helped you get through that six week stint in Kindred. While I got it, I also knew you couldn't go through that again.

As I said, this injury is devastating, and no one knows that better than you. It changes every aspect of your life and your personality. I know it has obviously changed your personality, but it has changed everyone who loves you as well.

I have to say that the little bit I do talk about the accident, occasionally someone will attempt to put a positive spin on it. Let me just say the essay I helped write for Jamie's assignment her first year of college is basically bull. There is little to nothing positive about this injury. So, when I heard, "I am sure the accident brought you and Trenton closer," I politely disagreed. I don't know, I may not have been that polite.

The 11th Anniversary

We just passed the 11th anniversary of your accident. I know it must be hard for you to believe, but it has taken me a year to compile my thoughts. If you read this, you may wonder how on earth it took me so long to finish this. Let me just say, this has not been easy for me. I overthink everything. This is not good when you are putting your thoughts on paper!

We've had several discussions about me writing this, but even more discussions about me publishing this. I am more compelled than ever to publish it for a couple of reasons. I was recently at a conference for work. During a lunch break there were a few of us chatting about the cost of health care. There was a man from the UK as well as two of my co-workers. One of the co-workers brought up Christopher Reeve, stating if her husband had an accident and was paralyzed she couldn't afford to take care of him.

I said, "I know you don't know this, but my son was in an accident and is now a quadriplegic." She didn't act like she heard me and continued to discuss the exorbitant amount of money it would take to sustain someone like Christopher Reeve. I know it doesn't sound like a big deal, but she clearly didn't care about my feelings. You don't end a life because you can't afford it, or it isn't what you expected, or what you bargained for in life.

And the second reason is, you chose to live.

Recently a book was released, ***Me Before You***, as well as a movie version of the book. I know I can't believe I read it either, but I thought the ending would be different. The book was a great story but I wanted the happy ending. You can have a happy ending and I don't believe anyone looking in can see that. I want people to know you are happy, you have family and friends who adore you and thank God every day you are here.

Today and moving forward...

So where are you now? You are slowly getting up in your chair more and stemming your muscles in the hopes of getting a nerve transplant procedure. The hope would be to get some functionality in your arms. I know how much you are hoping to get some use of your arms with this procedure and I pray it is successful.

Your health seems pretty good. Honestly, when you are in bed for so long, I think it is very similar to when you didn't eat for so long, and you didn't talk for so long. It is difficult to get back into even wanting to do that activity again.

Last summer for your birthday your dad and I got you a sip and puff fishing rod. You love to fish and you seemed to love it. Of course, I then thought I should move to a lake so you would have easy access. I had pretty much decided the layout of the deck so you could fish to your heart's content, but you squelched that idea very quickly. The first fish you caught was at your Dad's house, as they live on a lake. It was a good sized catfish. You told us we needed to clean it fairly quickly, so having never cleaned a fish, but having seen my parents clean a bunch, I thought to myself, "I've got this." But, just in case, I googled it. The first thing it said was to cut the tail off which would allow the fish to "bleed out" and die quickly and humanely. Let me tell you, there is nothing further from the truth. This was agony. All Cathy had was a kitchen knife so we (your dad and I) proceeded to try to filet this fish. About three minutes in I said to your Dad, "Lord, the things we have done for this kid," to which he agreed. Your Dad grew up on a farm and he knew less about cleaning fish than I did. Needless to say, we ended up with about a quarter size piece of fish. And, you immediately ordered a filet knife.

You have two very good caregivers you trust and like. You have Nancy for meals and daily needs. Thanks to Tyson and Sam, you can control your lights, heat, fans, blinds, television, and the list will continue to grow with the latest technology. For Christmas this year I got you Amazon's Alexa (a voice-activated device that cotrols lights, thermostat, plays music and reads audiobooks and news) and you have bought another one for the living room.

Your friends and family are just as amazing as they were in the beginning.

We have an annual golf tournament which benefits you and helps offset some costs. But, what you enjoy most is all the family and friends that come out for it. You love to see everyone and your speech at the end of the night is always heartfelt and hopeful.

Of course we have good moments and not-so-good moments. I know there is not a day that goes by we don't wish things were different for you. But, having said that and working at a pediatric hospital, I see and hear about many diseases, syndromes, conditions and disorders. They are each heartbreaking. I am and will always fight for the one that affects you. And, I will never stop hoping, praying and believing you will one day walk again.

Resources

Project Walk-Kansas City - Based in Overland Park, KS, Project Walk-Kansas City is a state-of-the-art spinal cord injury recovery center that is dedicated to meeting your recovery needs with up-to-date training techniques. We believe that traditional approaches to therapy can be further enhanced, allowing clients to get more out of our facility. Our approach, based on The Dardzinski Method, uses intense activity-based recovery, backed by research and technology to expose those affected by paralysis to the most forward-thinking rehabilitation in the industry. For more information visit: projectwalk-kansascity.org

Christopher and Dana Reeve Foundation and their NRN (Neurorecovery Network) - This is a great illustration of how far the idea, and possibility of SCI recovery has come in the last 5-10 years. https://www.christopherreeve.org/

Kennedy Krieger Hospital - They do amazing work with the use of electrical stimulation for paralysis recovery. https://www.kennedykrieger.org/

Restorative Therapies (they make electrical stimulation equipment). http://www.restorative-therapies.com/

Madonna Rehabilitation Hospital specializes in rehabilitation programs for traumatic brain injuries and spinal cord injuries as well as stroke and pulmonary conditions for children and adults. http://www.madonna.org/

Frazier Rehab – Research for Locomotor Training (LT) for recovery of function after SCI, or other causes of paralysis. They still do a big bulk of research with LT for recovery from paralysis. http://www.kentuckyonehealth.org/locomotor-training

Craig Hospital – World-renowned rehabilitation hospital specializing in the neuro-rehabilitation and research of patients with spinal cord injury and traumatic brain injury. https://craighospital.org/

Stowers Institute - A 10-acre research and educational facility in Kansas City that specializes in stem cell research and medical applications. Founded by Jim and Virginia Stowers, the first labs opened in November of 2000 with a mission of expanding understanding of the secrets of life and improving life's quality through innovative approaches to the causes, treatment and prevention of diseases. www.stowers.org

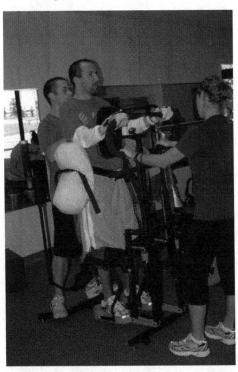

Staff at Craig placed a bear with the sip and puff straw by his mouth and a towel over his stomach while Trenton was in therapy. This is how Trenton laid in bed when he wasn't in therapy.

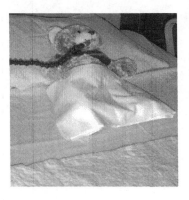

Project Walk--Standing for quads helps patients with their circulation, reduces muscle spasticity and lower extremity edema and helps with several other conditions.

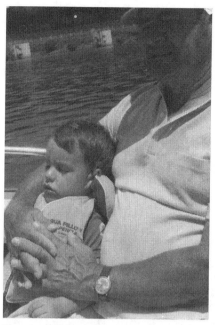

Trenton fell asleep on Grandpa Delmer while riding a boat at the lake.

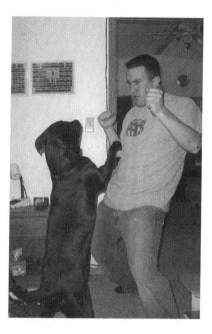

Trenton playing with his dog, "Willy."

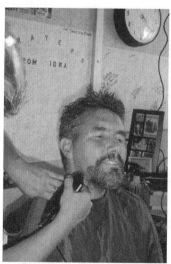

Rick getting his beard shaved because Trenton was, "Vent free."

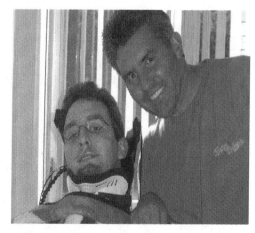

Rick and Trenton at Craig Hospital

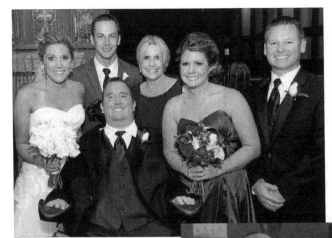

Jamie's wedding (left) and Trenton with nephew Liam. (Below)

(Below) Jamie's wedding, front row–Emma, Madi; 2nd row–Cathy, Rick, Jamie, Trenton and Ashley and back row–Chris, Chance and Blaise (who are Cathy's kids) and Tyson

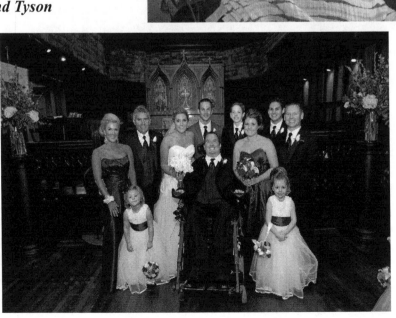

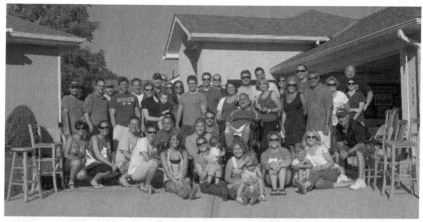

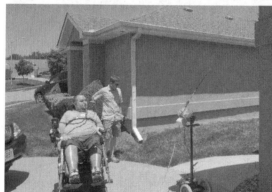

(Above) Trenton's 30th birthday party, attended by a few family members and friends.

(Left) Trenton with his new sip and puff fishing pole

The first fish he caught with his new fishing pole. Chance and Blaise are with him.

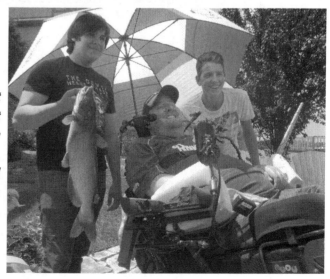

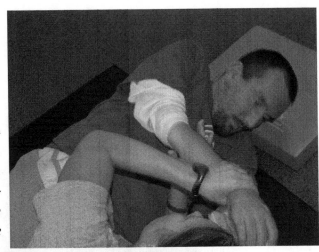

Project Walk staffers assist Trenton by positioning him for his next exercise

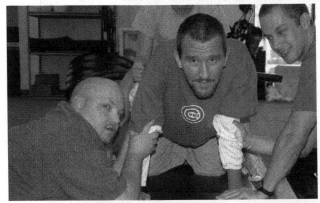

Staffer Denny, (left) and Susan's son-in-law Chris (right) during therapy at Project Walk and a closeup of the quad positioning (below)

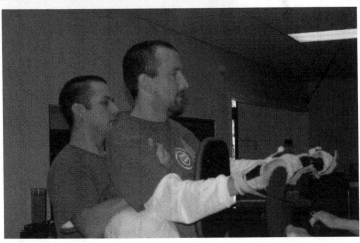

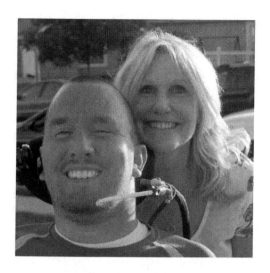

About the Author

This is Susan Baier's first book. While she has never written a book before, she is an avid reader and loves biographies and historical fiction. She has a bachelor's degree in Social Psychology from Park University in Parkville, Missouri. A native of Kansas City, Missouri, she was a stay-at-home mom for many years. She has been with Children's Mercy Hospital for nearly 13 years and seven of those years as a Patient Advocate. She is divorced; however, she and her ex-husband, Rick 1, remain good friends. She has been with Ric 2 for over 10 years.

Her passions include her family and friends . . . and now, spinal cord injury (SCI) awareness.

Susan spends her free time with her family and friends and loves to travel.

Besides residing with Ric 2, she has two golden doodles and two cats.